# Cultural Competence IN PATIENT CARE

Dianne McAdams-Jones

innovativeink
PUBLISHING
A Division of Kendall Hunt

Cover image Shutterstock.com

innovative ink PUBLISHING
A Division of Kendall Hunt

www.innovativeinkpublishing.com
*Send all inquiries to*:
4050 Westmark Drive
Dubuque, IA 52004-1840



Print ISBN: 979-8-3197-4318-3
eBook ISBN: 979-8-3197-4319-0



Published in the United States of America

# Contents

# Preface

The history of healthcare is deeply intertwined with the evolution of healthcare ethics, science, and social policy. Among the most sobering chapters in this history is the era of eugenics—a movement that sought to improve the genetic quality of human populations through selective breeding and, in many cases, coercive measures. While eugenics is often associated with early-20th-century policies and atrocities, its influence on healthcare practices and public health initiatives remains a critical area of reflection for healthcare professionals today. Understanding this context is not merely an academic exercise; it is an ethical imperative that shapes how healthcare professionals approach patient care, advocacy, and social justice.

Eugenics emerged during a time of rapid scientific advancement and societal change, when concepts of heredity and genetics were misunderstood and misapplied. Health professionals, including nurses, were often enlisted to implement policies such as forced sterilizations, institutionalization, and discriminatory healthcare practices targeting marginalized populations. These actions were justified under the guise of "improving public health," yet they inflicted profound harm, violating human rights and perpetuating systemic inequities. For healthcare, this history underscores the importance of critically examining the ethical foundations of their practice and recognizing how societal biases can infiltrate healthcare systems.

Even today, the echoes of eugenics persist in subtle but significant ways. Discussions about genetic screening, reproductive technologies, and health disparities raise questions about autonomy, consent, and equity. Healthcare workers and professionals must be vigilant in ensuring that advancements in genetics and personalized medicine do not replicate the discriminatory ideologies of the past. This requires a deep understanding of the historical context of eugenics, its impact on vulnerable populations, othering, and the lessons it offers for contemporary practice.

# Introduction to the Concept of Ethics in Healthcare Practice

Ethics in healthcare is the cornerstone of professional practice, guiding all professionals in making decisions that uphold patient dignity, autonomy, and well-being. Rooted in principles such as beneficence, nonmaleficence, justice, and respect for persons, healthcare ethics ensures that care is delivered with compassion and integrity. Healthcare professionals often face complex situations where clinical judgment intersects with moral responsibility—such as end-of-life care, informed consent, and resource allocation. In these moments, ethical frameworks provide clarity and direction.

Central to professional ethics is the commitment to **advocacy**. Healthcare professionals serve as patient advocates, safeguarding rights and ensuring that individuals receive equitable, respectful care regardless of socioeconomic status, cultural background, or health condition. Confidentiality and privacy are equally vital, requiring healthcare professionals to protect sensitive information while fostering trust in the healthcare professional–patient relationship.

Modern healthcare introduces new ethical challenges, including genetic testing, technological interventions, and disparities in access to care. Healthcare professionals must balance innovation with humanity, ensuring that advancements do not compromise ethical standards. Continuous education in ethics empowers healthcare professionals to navigate these dilemmas thoughtfully and uphold professional codes, such as those outlined by the American Nurses Association (ANA), the American Association of Respiratory Care, the American Occupational Therapy Association, the American Physical Therapy Association, the American Medical Association, the American Association of Colleges of Nursing, to name a few.

Ultimately, ethics in healthcare is not static; it evolves with societal values and medical progress. By embracing ethical principles, healthcare providers affirm their role as compassionate caregivers and moral agents, committed to promoting health, preventing harm, and advocating for justice in every aspect of patient care.

**Purpose**: The author wrote this short book of historical reflection and program planning for educators as a means of support for healthcare professionals struggling to teach and connect past historical harms that affect today's practice. This book offers examples of how to prepare a healthcare lesson on past medical and healthcare harm because some educators have exclaimed, "I would include it, but I don't know how I can fit it into my curriculum."

**Aim**: The aim of this book is to provide examples of how to comfortably include difficult healthcare inclusive topics into a curriculum. This book is for all healthcare providers!

# Convening and Artificial Intelligence Advisory Board of Health Professionals

A dear colleague and friend suggested I convene an advisory board on health, education and equity by way of generative artificial intelligence (conversation with Dr. Alaa Alsarhan, March, 2026). An AI (Artificial Intelligence) Advisory Board would serve as the foundation and the framework from which to develop valuable insights from experienced healthcare professionals, directing the focus and navigating the structure of this book. The board could include the views of stakeholders, promoting a unified approach to healthcare delivery and innovation. Furthermore, the advisory board would include clinical realities and regulatory standards, enhancing the overall effectiveness of information provided in this book for the education of healthcare professionals. The prompt given for AI was to explore the links provided from AACN (American Association of Colleges of Nursing), the NLN (National League for Nursing), the AMA (American Medical Association), the American Occupational Therapy Association (AOTA), the American Physical Therapy Association (APTA), the Physician Assistant Education Association (PAEA), the American Association of Respiratory Care (AARC), and the American Nurses Association (ANA) and then write 1,000 words about how each organization approached equity relative to eugenics in their practice. Once this information was generated, I asked for references and a comparison and contrast between and over all of the organizations. I used the latter to create the introduction, here, and highlighted each organization going forward. I cross-referenced and checked the information provided by AI and wrote the conclusion.

The harmful legacy of eugenics in medicine underscores the importance of ethical vigilance in healthcare. By promoting discrimination, violating autonomy, and distorting scientific practice, eugenics caused widespread harm that continues to shape health disparities and trust in medical institutions. However, the healthcare professions have taken decisive steps to confront this past and build a more just and inclusive future.

Frameworks such as the *ANA Code of Ethics*, along with stated positions from the NLN, AMA, AACN, and other organizations, demonstrate a clear commitment to rejecting eugenic principles. By emphasizing dignity, equity, patient autonomy, and social justice, modern healthcare redefines its role as a partner in promoting well-being rather than a gatekeeper of genetic "fitness."

This ongoing transformation requires continued reflection, education, and reform. As new technologies emerge and societal challenges evolve, healthcare professionals must remain grounded in ethical principles that affirm the value of every human life. In doing so, the profession not only moves away from the shadows of eugenics but also advances toward a more compassionate and equitable system of care.

Healthcare professions today are actively transforming themselves through strong ethical frameworks and position statements that confront past injustices and promote inclusive, patient-centered care. Organizations such as the American Association for Respiratory Care (AARC), the American Occupational Therapy Association (AOTA), the American Physical Therapy Association (APTA), and the Physician Assistant Education Association/American Academy of Physician Associates (PAEA/AAPA) play a central role in guiding this change. Furthermore, the American Nurses Association (ANA), the National League for Nurses (NLN), the American Medical Association (AMA), and the American Association of Colleges of Nursing (AACN) add sentiment in unison. Their codes of ethics and professional guidelines reflect a collective reckoning with historical harms—including the legacy of eugenics in medicine—and an intentional effort to reshape professional values toward equity, dignity, and social responsibility.

## ACKNOWLEDGING HISTORY AND ITS IMPACT

The transformation of healthcare professions begins with acknowledging the historical role of medicine in supporting harmful ideologies such as eugenics. The American Medical Association's exploration of physicians' involvement in the eugenics movement highlights how healthcare professionals once participated in discriminatory practices, including forced sterilization and the marginalization of individuals based on perceived genetic "fitness." This history demonstrates how professional authority was misused to justify inequity and harm.

Modern organizations use this historical awareness as a foundation for change. By explicitly recognizing past ethical failures, they create space for accountability and reform. This acknowledgment also reinforces the importance of ethical vigilance—ensuring that emerging practices and technologies do not replicate similar injustices under new forms.

## PROMOTING DIVERSITY AND INCLUSION IN RESPIRATORY CARE

The American Association for Respiratory Care's (AARC, n.d. and 2017) Position Statement on Diversity and Inclusion exemplifies how professional organizations actively address inequity in healthcare. The AARC, 2017, emphasizes that diversity strengthens the profession and improves patient outcomes by ensuring culturally responsive care. It calls for the recruitment and retention of a diverse workforce, equitable treatment of patients, and the elimination of systemic barriers within healthcare systems.

This position reflects a clear departure from exclusionary ideologies such as eugenics. Rather than viewing human differences as deficits, the AARC reframes diversity as a strength. The organization's commitment to inclusion fosters an environment where patients are respected as individuals with unique backgrounds, and where practitioners are trained to recognize and address health disparities rather than perpetuate them.

## ETHICAL RECKONING AND THE SHIFT IN MEDICINE

Modern medical ethics represents a conscious effort to confront and move away from this legacy. The American Medical Association (AMA, n.d.) has acknowledged the profession's role in historical injustices and emphasized the need for accountability and reform. In discussions of genome editing (O'Reilly, 2017), the AMA underscores that emerging technologies must be guided by ethical principles that prioritize patient welfare, informed consent, and social justice. While genetic interventions hold promise for treating disease, the ethical framework explicitly cautions against applications that echo eugenic goals, such as selecting traits based on subjective notions of desirability, prioritizing biased assumptions over evidence, and embedding race and genetics into clinical decision-making in such harmful ways. The continued critique of race-based clinical algorithms—such as race-adjusted pulmonary function tests—illustrates how remnants of eugenic thinking persisted well into modern medicine. The American Thoracic Society and related organizations have explicitly called for reevaluation of such practices, recognizing that race is a social construct rather than a biological determinant and that its misuse can exacerbate inequities.

The American Medical Association apologized to the Black physicians relative to the discrimination imposed upon them by the profession; it was offered as a foundation for the profession to begin its healing (AMA, 2021 & Madera, 2021). This shift reflects a broader transformation in how healthcare defines its mission. Instead of controlling or improving populations, contemporary medicine focuses on supporting individuals' health and autonomy. Ethical guidelines emphasize respect for persons, beneficence, nonmaleficence, and justice—principles that directly counter the coercive and discriminatory practices of eugenics.

## OCCUPATIONAL THERAPY AND HOLISTIC ETHICAL PRACTICE

The American Occupational Therapy (AOTA) *Code of ethics* (2025) further illustrates how professional standards guide transformative change. Occupational therapy emphasizes holistic care, focusing on individuals' ability to participate meaningfully in daily life. Its ethical code promotes principles such as beneficence, nonmaleficence, autonomy, justice, veracity, and fidelity.

Particularly significant is the emphasis on *justice*, which requires practitioners to provide equitable services and challenge discrimination. This principle directly counters the discriminatory practices historically associated with eugenics. Occupational therapists are encouraged to advocate for underserved populations, address systemic inequities, and ensure that all individuals have access to opportunities that support health and well-being.

Additionally, the focus on autonomy respects each patient's right to make decisions about their own life and care. This stands in stark contrast to eugenic practices, which often stripped individuals of their agency. Through these ethical commitments, the AOTA fosters a profession grounded in respect, empowerment, and inclusivity.

## THE ANA CODE OF ETHICS: EDUCATION, DIVERSITY, AND INCLUSION IN HEALTHCARE

The move away from eugenics is further reinforced through educational and institutional reforms. The American Nurses Association (ANA, n.d.-a) emphasizes diversity, equity, and inclusion as essential components of nursing education. By preparing healthcare professionals to understand cultural, social, and structural determinants of health, these initiatives counteract the reductionist and biased perspectives of eugenics.

Incorporating social determinants of health into curricula—such as housing, income, education, and systemic racism—shifts the focus from blaming individuals or their genetics to addressing broader societal factors (ANA, n.d.-b). This approach aligns with ethical care and promotes more accurate, equitable clinical decision-making.

## PHYSICAL THERAPY AND RESPECT FOR HUMAN DIGNITY

The American Physical Therapy Association's Code of Ethics, n.d., also plays a vital role in guiding professional change. It highlights the physical therapist's responsibility to respect the inherent dignity and rights of all individuals. Core principles include accountability, compassion, integrity, and social responsibility.

A key aspect of the APTA code, n.d., is its recognition of the therapist's role in addressing health disparities and advocating for patients. Physical therapists are expected to provide care without discrimination and to actively work toward improving access to services. This aligns with a broader movement in healthcare that shifts focus from biological determinism to social determinants of health.

By embedding these values into professional conduct, the APTA ensures that practitioners move away from reductionist and hierarchical views of human worth. Instead, care is individualized and grounded in respect for each patient's unique experiences and needs.

## NATIONAL LEAGUE FOR NURSES: PROFESSIONAL CONDUCT OF THE NURSE

The National League for Nursing (NLN) takes a strong ethical stance that both implicitly rejects eugenics and actively promotes equity in healthcare and nursing education. Although the NLN does not explicitly name eugenics in its position statements, its ethical principles fundamentally oppose the ideology's core beliefs, particularly the notion that some individuals have greater worth than others based on genetic or social characteristics.

Central to the NLN's position is its emphasis on *human dignity and justice* (NLN, n.d.-a). The Ethical Principles for Nursing Education affirm that all individuals possess inherent worth and must be treated with respect and fairness. This directly contradicts eugenic thinking, which historically justified discrimination, exclusion, and coercive practices such as forced sterilization. The NLN's commitment to *autonomy* further reinforces this stance, emphasizing patients' and learners' rights to make decisions about their own lives without coercion.

In addition to rejecting discriminatory ideologies, the NLN strongly advocates for *equity and inclusion* (NLN, n.d.-b). Its vision statement on achieving diversity and meaningful inclusion highlights the importance of creating a nursing workforce that reflects the populations it serves. The NLN calls for systemic changes in education, including removing barriers to entry, promoting cultural competence, and addressing social determinants of health.

Ultimately, the NLN positions nursing as a profession grounded in *social justice and ethical responsibility* (NLN, n.d.-c). By centering dignity, equity, and inclusion, the organization not only distances itself from the legacy of eugenics but also actively works to build a more just and equitable healthcare system.

## AMERICAN ASSOCIATION OF COLLEGES OF NURSING: DIVERSITY IS ESSENTIAL TO EXCELLENCE IN NURSING EDUCATION AND HEALTHCARE DELIVERY

Rather than viewing differences as deficits, the American Association of Colleges of Nursing (AACN) n.d. recognizes that varied backgrounds, experiences, and perspectives strengthen clinical practice and improve patient outcomes. This approach stands in contrast to eugenic ideologies that sought to control or limit human variation. By promoting a diverse nursing workforce, the AACN supports more culturally competent care and helps address longstanding disparities in health outcomes among marginalized populations.

Equally important is AACN's focus on *equity and social determinants of health* (AACN, n.d.). The organization emphasizes that health disparities are rooted not in biology but, instead, in systemic inequities such as access to education, economic stability, and structural racism. This perspective directly challenges the biological determinism that underpinned eugenic thinking. AACN calls for nursing education to prepare professionals who can recognize and address these broader influences on health (AACN, n.d.).

Ultimately, AACN positions nurses as *advocates for social justice and health equity*. Through inclusive education, ethical leadership, and a commitment to fairness, the organization is helping transform healthcare into a system that values all individuals equally and works to eliminate discrimination in all forms (AACN, n.d.).

## ETHICAL CONDUCT IN THE PHYSICIAN ASSISTANT PROFESSION

The Guidelines for Ethical Conduct for the Physician Assistant (PA) profession reinforce similar principles within the PA field. These guidelines emphasize patient autonomy, beneficence, nonmaleficence, and justice, while also addressing the importance of cultural competence and professional integrity, (PAEA, 2021).

Physician assistants, 2021, are expected to develop trusting relationships with patients, respect diverse backgrounds, and advocate for equitable care. The guidelines also highlight the responsibility to challenge unethical behavior and systemic inequities within healthcare systems. This advocacy role is critical in driving change at both individual and institutional levels.

The PA profession's emphasis on teamwork and collaboration further supports equitable care. By working across disciplines and engaging with patients as partners, physician assistants contribute to a healthcare environment that values inclusion and shared decision-making.

Furthermore, continued reflection on historical injustices ensures that the lessons of the past remain relevant. As new technologies such as genetic editing emerge, ethical frameworks must adapt to address potential risks while promoting beneficial innovation.

In conclusion,

**This short book will illuminate historical context developing lesson plans embracing cultural competency on the following topics.**

## Skin pigmentation...can change how we approach healthcare.

Skin color is more than a superficial characteristic—it can significantly influence diagnosis, treatment, and recovery in healthcare. Variations in pigmentation often affect how certain conditions present clinically, which can lead to disparities in care if providers are not adequately trained to recognize these differences. For example, pressure injuries, rashes, and cyanosis may appear less obvious on darker skin tones, increasing the risk of delayed diagnosis and complications. Similarly, jaundice and pallor are traditionally assessed through visual cues that may not be as apparent in patients with richly pigmented skin, requiring alternative assessment strategies.

Beyond diagnosis, skin color can impact treatment outcomes. Melanin levels influence responses to certain dermatologic treatments, such as laser therapy or chemical peels, where inappropriate settings can cause hyperpigmentation or scarring in darker skin. Additionally, cultural and genetic factors associated with skin color may affect wound healing, susceptibility to keloids, and tolerance to medications.

Recovery is also shaped by systemic inequities. Patients with darker skin tones often face implicit bias and structural barriers that limit access to timely, culturally competent care. Healthcare professionals play a critical role in mitigating these disparities by adopting inclusive assessment techniques, advocating for equitable treatment, and educating themselves about skin tone variations in clinical presentations.

Understanding these nuances is essential for delivering safe, effective, and respectful care. By recognizing how skin color influences health outcomes, nurses can ensure that all patients receive accurate diagnoses and optimal recovery pathways.

## Healthcare as a Right or a Privilege

The debate over whether healthcare is a right or a privilege lies at the heart of health policy and ethics. Viewing healthcare as a **right** means that every individual, regardless of income, social status, or circumstance, is entitled to access essential medical services. This perspective is grounded in principles of human dignity and social justice, asserting that health is fundamental to life and well-being. Advocates argue that denying care based on ability to pay perpetuates inequality and undermines public health, as untreated illness can lead to widespread societal consequences.

Conversely, considering healthcare a **privilege** frames it as a benefit earned through personal responsibility and financial contribution. Supporters of this view emphasize limited resources and the need for sustainability, arguing that individuals should share in the cost of care to prevent overuse and maintain system viability. They contend that making healthcare universally free or guaranteed could strain budgets and reduce incentives for healthy behaviors.

This debate is not merely theoretical—it shapes policies on insurance coverage, government programs, and access to life-saving treatments. For nurses and health professionals, understanding both perspectives is crucial for advocacy and ethical decision-making. While the tension between rights and privileges persists, most agree that a balance must be struck ensuring equitable access while promoting accountability and resource stewardship.

Ultimately, how society answers this question reflects its values—whether prioritizing collective responsibility for health or individual autonomy in managing care.

## The Controversy Over Those Who Can or Cannot Contribute Financially to Their Own Healthcare

The question of whether individuals who cannot contribute financially to their healthcare should still receive medical services is one of the most polarizing issues in health policy and ethics. On one side, advocates for universal healthcare argue that access to health services is a basic human right, essential for preserving life and dignity. They emphasize that illness does not discriminate based on income, and withholding care from those unable to pay can lead to preventable suffering, public health crises, and deepening social inequities. From this perspective, healthcare systems should prioritize compassion and collective responsibility over financial capability.

Conversely, critics contend that healthcare resources are finite and must be distributed responsibly. They argue that requiring individuals to contribute financially promotes accountability and sustainability, preventing overuse and reducing strain on public systems. Opponents fear that offering free care without contribution could encourage dependency and undermine incentives for personal responsibility, ultimately jeopardizing the viability of healthcare infrastructure.

This controversy is further complicated by structural barriers—such as unemployment, disability, and systemic discrimination—that limit some individuals' ability to pay. Ethical considerations demand that these factors be weighed carefully, as denying care based solely on financial status can perpetuate injustice.

Ultimately, the debate reflects a tension between two values: equity and sustainability. Resolving it requires nuanced policies that balance compassion with practicality, ensuring that healthcare remains accessible while maintaining the integrity of the system.

## The Concept of Eugenics Situating Health Professions as Ethical

The history of eugenics presents a profound ethical challenge for healthcare, highlighting the importance of moral accountability in healthcare. During the early 20th century, eugenics—promoting selective breeding and sterilization to "improve" human populations—was widely accepted in scientific and medical communities. Nurses were often tasked with implementing these policies, including involuntary sterilizations and institutionalization of individuals deemed "unfit." These actions, justified under the guise of public health, violated fundamental human rights and inflicted lasting harm on vulnerable populations.

This historical context situates healthcare as an ethical profession by underscoring the need for vigilance against discriminatory ideologies. Modern healthcare is grounded in principles of autonomy, beneficence, and justice, ensuring that care respects individual dignity and informed consent. Understanding the legacy of eugenics reminds us all that ethical practice is not static; it requires continuous reflection and advocacy to prevent the resurgence of harmful biases in contemporary healthcare.

Today, advancements in genetics and reproductive technologies pose new ethical dilemmas. Healthcare professionals must ensure that these innovations do not replicate eugenic thinking, particularly in decisions about genetic screening or selective reproduction. By embracing cultural humility, promoting equity, and safeguarding patient rights, nurses affirm their role as moral agents committed to compassionate, inclusive care.

The lessons of eugenics are clear: Ethical healthcare demands courage to challenge injustice and a steadfast commitment to human dignity. This responsibility defines healthcare not only as a science but also as a profession rooted in ethics.

## Supporting the Health of Others Who Are Not Like You

Healthcare is a profession built on compassion, equity, and respect for human dignity. One of its core ethical principles is providing care without prejudice, regardless of a patient's background, beliefs, or identity. Supporting the health of individuals who are different from oneself—whether in culture, language, socioeconomic status, or lifestyle—is not optional; it is fundamental to professional integrity and quality care.

Patients come from diverse backgrounds, and these differences often influence health behaviors, access to care, and treatment outcomes. Healthcare professionals must recognize that personal biases, even unconscious ones, can affect clinical judgment and patient interactions. By actively embracing diversity, healthcare professionals foster trust, improve communication, and ensure that care plans are culturally sensitive and patient centered.

Moreover, health disparities disproportionately affect marginalized populations and outcomes are less than desirable. Healthcare professionals have a responsibility to advocate for equity, addressing barriers such as discrimination, poverty, and limited health literacy. Supporting those who are "not like you" means listening without judgment, respecting autonomy, and tailoring interventions to meet unique needs.

Ultimately, healthcare is not about similarity—it is about humanity. Every patient deserves compassionate, competent care, regardless of differences. By committing to inclusivity and empathy, healthcare professionals uphold the highest ethical standards and contribute to a healthcare system that values all lives equally.

## Division Community Conversations About Race and Race Behavior

If communities actively engaged in conversations about race and race-related behaviors, the landscape of social interaction and health equity would look profoundly different. These dialogues would create spaces for honesty, empathy, and education, dismantling misconceptions and reducing prejudice. Community forums, schools, and healthcare settings could serve as platforms where individuals share lived experiences, explore historical contexts, and confront implicit biases. Such conversations would not be accusatory, but, instead, they would be collaborative, fostering mutual respect and understanding (Fairbanks, 2015).

In practice, these discussions would normalize diversity and highlight the systemic factors that shape racial behaviors, such as cultural traditions, socioeconomic disparities, and historical injustices fueling social learning. Communities would learn to distinguish between cultural differences and harmful stereotypes, promoting inclusivity rather than division. Healthcare professionals would benefit greatly from these conversations, as they would enhance cultural competence and improve patient outcomes by addressing disparities rooted in race.

Moreover, these dialogues would empower marginalized voices, ensuring that policies and practices reflect equity and justice. Schools and workplaces could integrate structured programs, similar to the ones offered in this book, that teach critical thinking about race, encouraging individuals to challenge discriminatory behaviors and advocate for fairness.

Ultimately, communities that embrace these conversations would become more cohesive, resilient, and compassionate with better healthcare outcomes thus decreasing reentry for same health problem. Understanding race and race behavior is not about erasing differences; rather, it is about valuing them—creating a society where diversity is celebrated and equality is a shared responsibility.

## References

Alsarhan, Alaa. Conversation March 2026 relative to equity from the lens of an AI generated advisory board on equity relative to cultural competence. Dr. Alsarhan is the Director of Academic Analytics at Utah Valley University. Co-founder of Horizon Analytics LLC. Co-inventor of SEGO Engagement tool. https://www.linkedin.com/in/alaa-alsarhanphd/

American Association of Colleges of Nursing. (n.d.). *Position statement* (under revision). https://www.aacnnursing.org/portals/42/news/position-statements/diversity-inclusion.pdf

American Association of Respiratory Care. (n.d.). *Position statement on diversity and inclusion.* https://www.aarc.org/wp-content/uploads/documents/statement-of-diversity-and-Inclusion.pdf

American Association of Respiratory Care. (2017). *Statement of ethics and professional conduct.* https://www.aarc.org/wp-content/uploads/2017/03/statement-of-ethics.pdf

American Association of Respiratory Care. (2023). *American Thoracic Society issues new statement on race, ethnicity and PFTs.* https://www.aarc.org/news/041723-rcc/

American Nurses Association. (n.d.-a). *Code of ethics.* https://codeofethics.ana.org/provisions

American Nurses Association. (n.d.-b). *Our racial reckoning statement.* https://www.nursingworld.org/practice-policy/workforce/racism-in-nursing/RacialReckoningStatement/

American Occupational Therapy Association. (2025). *Occupational therapy code of ethics. American Journal of Occupational Therapy, 79*(Suppl. 3). https://research.aota.org/ajot/article/79/Supplement%203/7913060400/28485/AOTA-2025-Occupational-Therapy-Code-of-Ethics

American Physical Therapy Association. (n.d.). *Code of ethics for the physical therapist.* https://www.apta.org/siteassets/pdfs/policies/code-of-ethics-for-the-physical-therapist.pdf

Fairbanks, D. J. (2015). *Everyone is African: How science explodes the myth of race.* Prometheus Books.

Madera, J. (2021). *Reckoning with medicine's history of racism.* https://www.ama-assn.org/about/leadership/reckoning-medicine-s-history-racism

National League for Nursing. (n.d.-a). *Achieving diversity and meaningful inclusion in nursing education.* https://www.nln.org/docs/default-source/uploadedfiles/professional-development-programs/vision-statement-achieving-diversity.pdf

National League for Nursing. (n.d.-b). *Diversity and inclusion.* https://www.nln.org/public-policy/nursing-education-issues/diversity

National League for Nursing. (n.d.-c). *Ethical principles for nursing education.* https://www.nln.org/docs/default-source/uploadedfiles/default-document-library/ethical-principles-for-nursing-education-final-final-010312.pdf?sfvrsn=4b49d00d_0

O'Reilly, K. B. (2017, August 4). *Genome editing and the AMA Code of Medical Ethics.* https://www.ama-assn.org/about/ethics/genome-editing-and-ama-code-medical-ethics

Physician Assistant Education Association. (2021). *Guidelines for ethical conduct for the PA profession.* https://www.aapa.org/wp-content/uploads/2021/11/Guidelines-for-Ethical-Conduct-for-the-PA-Profession-7-1-21.pdf

The American Medical Association: The History of Physicians and the American Eugenics Movement. (n.d.). https://edhub.ama-assn.org/science-medicine-public-health/audio-player/18862697

# Skin

## LESSON OBJECTIVES

Upon completion of this lesson, the student will:

a. Identify two common disease presentations or skin abnormalities (such as erythema, cyanosis, jaundice, and infection) on light and dark skin.
b. Discuss how different skin abnormalities manifest on light versus dark skin tones.
c. Apply appropriate assessment techniques to ensure equitable and accurate clinical evaluation on light and dark skin

## INTRODUCTION

Bedside healthcare providers are often one of the first providers to see the patient and, then, one of the last providers to see the patient. The purpose of this lesson is to bring an awareness to possible assessment inequities that may arise when healthcare providers are taught focusing on one skin type. Then nurses often have some of the most intimate conversations with the patient; hence, they could be said to be the most trusted person in the patient's circle. According to a publication at Johns Hopkins University (January 17, 2025), nurses consistently are ranked #1 as the most trusted by the patient. In that space, as nurses and healthcare providers, we must continue to situate our best efforts for the patient's interest. That would include learning as much about all our "types" of patients as we possibly can. Science is always evolving, and so, for us, as a people, our life circumstances change, too, in tandem; as healthcare professionals, we must meet those challenges where the patient is positioned (DiStefano, 2025). As the most trusted, we should be the most trustworthy and provide the most equitable care.

## SKIN

One of the first things we see when a person approaches us is the skin. Why? Because it is the largest organ of the body, and, according to much of the medical literature, it covers approximately 98–100% of the body's surface. Of course, then, the color of the skin becomes the next likely thing seen as a prominent descriptor of the person. Color of the skin is significant if you are involved in caring for that person; as a health professional, this is important to notice. Not all diseases or skin reactions to diseases and the environment are similar between dark and light skin. A big reason for this is the physiology of the skin, particularly, ethnic skin (skin with color/melanin). Cole et al. (n.d.) give us an understanding of the meaning of melanocytes; essentially, melanocytes have a similar quantity in both dark- and light-skinned people. The difference here is, the melanocytes in the darker skin will produce more melanin. To avoid further harm to the patient's skin or a misdiagnosis, the healthcare professional would need to understand what this implies.

Be sure to use all senses during the assessment: look, listen, feel (palpate), and smell. Why? Darker skin may look ashen-colored, purplish, grey, or white when it is oxygen-deprived versus the tinted bluish color typically discussed in academic books. It is always better to look inside the patient's oral cavity examining the buccal mucosa for bluish color (decreased oxygenation) or pink color (adequate oxygenation) when assessing oxygenation.

Erythema and cyanosis are a lot harder to detect on darker skin; thus, the healthcare provider must rely on palpation and mucus membrane visualization during the assessment. Darker skin has a higher incidence of keloid formation due to hyper melanin production along with collagen overproduction. Increased melanin production in darker skin contributes to post-inflammatory hyperpigmentation. Bottom line—darker skin and lighter skin look very different when they manifest abnormalities.

Think about this: If the skin is producing more melanin, it tends to respond to an injury with a more exaggerated, perhaps labile response. This is manifested in scarring and even hyperpigmentation (Cole et al., 2009). With these facts in the mirror, as healthcare professionals we want to be certain to take the pigmentation and its various reactive genetic properties into our assessment. First, look carefully at the skin on admission and then make a note of every lump, bump, opening, scar, raised area, discolored area, freckled or spotted area, and any sighting that does not look normal. Then, hold a dialogue with the patient about the areas you have documented using any standard skin assessment guide, particularly discussing color (red, pale, bluish, grey, erythema, yellow eyes or yellow palm of hands), texture (smooth, rough, thin, or thick), turgor (elastic tone vs. non elastic tone, dehydrated), integrity (swelling, lesion, breaks in skin, cracked skin, a wound, a rash, a mole [raised or flat], a bruise [greenish or blackish color]), and temperature (warm, dry, cool, cold). While examining the skin over the entire body, be sure to ask the patient questions about their knowledge of your finding and when they noticed the finding and whether the finding has evolved since their first recognition. Darker skin would need a closer examination because the darkness cannot be assumed as normal, as the skin could be slightly darker than the other skin pointing to disease or trauma. So, in assessing darker skin, remember that darker skin is more reactive to surface trauma due to their melanocytes producing more melanin. Subsequently, the skin may turn gray, ashen, and paler during cyanosis, and the palms of the hands may turn yellow versus the eyes during liver disease (Cole et al., 2009). Often the patient is the best co-assessor because they often will have known of a skin change but tried many remedies to no avail attempting to address the skin change. This is dangerous; thus, questions such as—"How long do you recall this?"; "How long the skin has been looking like this?"; "Have you used any medicines on the skin?"; "What does your skin look like to you?"—are especially relevant.

## Why Is This Important?

So why is any of this important? This is important because it is possible to misidentify a skin condition if you are not familiar with a skin type. Also, personal perceptions about a type of people can cause health professionals to allow bias to interfere with their ability to implement best practices in the care of patients. Furthermore, a healthcare professional's thinking about color of skin relative to healthcare as a right or a privilege can play a role in how care is delivered.

The U.S. Department of Health and Human Services (n.d.-a and nd.-b) explains the framework of Social Determinants of Health and how this framework articulates in society with deep-rooted origins and long-lasting effects. It further reported from years of research that people of color are less likely to access or finish degrees in higher education and this, in turn, closes the door on getting opportunities to develop skills critical to access better-paying jobs that can change their economical and health outcomes (n.d.-a and n.d.-b). It also affects their ability to acquire private health insurance that many Americans access at a reasonable expense through their employment. This forces people of color to resort to the only method of care available through public assistance. As these people present to the healthcare system, the view from healthcare providers might be less than favorable.

At a western university a number of healthcare hopefuls were queried if healthcare was a right or a privilege. Qualitative design was used with a survey developed and critiqued by expert faculty from nursing; no survey was currently in existence. No psychometrics were performed; thus, this is a survey and not a research tool. Purposive sample was selected by university Institutional Research team providing emails for nurses and science majors. A Qualtrics survey was distributed. The data collected were coded and themed. The Institutional Review Board cleared the study. The research revealed,

*Healthcare Is a Right*

Just under 50% answered in the affirmative and the remaining answered in the negative. Another 11 respondents chose to provide a narrative and all narratives reported here are as they were reported in the survey. One respondent offered—"It's not a right, nobody deserves healthcare but as affluent as a nation as we are, we should guarantee everyone healthcare simply because we can. It's the mentality of giving 'someone else' healthcare rather than one of 'us' that's the problem. We could all be on the same team if people could just stop being awful selfish monsters." More respondents answered, "Yes, health should be a constitutional right"; "rights are things that don't force other people to be your slaves. If you have a right to healthcare that means you have a right to enslave others to pay for it"; "I believe it is a right, but if you don't need to pay for it or wish to not have medical insurance that is your prerogative and personal right. Therefore you should be punished by have fines brought against one's self in tax penalties"; "Because [it] benefits the poor"; "I believe everyone had a right to ACCESS to healthcare"; "I believe very basic healthcare should be [a] right"; "It should be available to everyone at not such a ridiculous cost, but I don't think it should just be free either"; "I believe that everyone should be able to have a form of healthcare available to them; regardless, however, I think that it's wrong that people take advantage of the fact that people of a higher financial status are paying for the healthcare for those who cannot provide for themselves. I think that the healthcare system provided through taxes of others should be used for those who really need it. Not those who take advantage, but on the other hand, identifying those types of people is not an easy task." "It's a right for people that live under the basic necessities, but not for the ones who take advantage."

I asked generative AI to assist with this analysis. According to generative AI's assistance with analyzing these responses, and the author agrees, generative AI summarized that those who supported healthcare as a right seemed to lean into moral and humanitarian grounds. On this question of healthcare being a right the narratives supported healthcare as a right arguing that healthcare should be universally accessible because it benefits society, especially the vulnerable. This includes references to the poor, individuals lacking basic necessities, and ensuring fairness. Others arguing against healthcare as a right make a point that healthcare is not inherently a right, emphasizing personal responsibility and concerns about economic consequences. Philosophically, some argue that labeling healthcare a right might infringe on others' freedom, such as forcing them to pay for others' healthcare. This perspective frames mandatory healthcare as equivalent to financial coercion. They offered, "Rights are things that don't force other people to be your slaves" and "If you have a right to healthcare, that means you have a right to enslave others to pay for it." There were definite tensions between rights and resources against moral arguments and practicality. Despite differences, most agree on the importance of ensuring access to healthcare, but with varying views on how and to what extent this should be achieved (McAdams-Jones and Sharp, 2026).

### *Healthcare Is a Privilege*

When the question was posed as a privilege, six of those surveyed responded in a narrative, and the percentages were roughly equally divided. The six narratives follow and are reported here as they were reported in the survey: "For the same reason above, not really? It shouldn't be seen as though one individual is getting a privilege from the country so much as we're taking care of ourselves by helping ourselves"; "No. Everyone deserves to be healthy"; "You earn it, you get it"; "It's not"; "Improved healthcare is with money to pay for it"; "Money should not be the reason that some people get healthcare and others do not. It is a necessity, regardless of one's financial situation."

Generative AI was tapped for help analyzing the responses. Close to those who answered in the affirmative (28 of them), 27 respondents argue against the idea of healthcare as a privilege. The moral imperative leaned on some who emphasize that health is a basic necessity and everyone deserves access to it, regardless of financial status or contributions. This was supported in responses such as "No. Everyone deserves to be healthy." Then, there was the collective responsibility that healthcare is about mutual care and self-preservation as a society, rather than viewing it as a privilege reserved for some. A supportive response to this belief was offered—"It shouldn't be seen as though one individual is getting a privilege from the country so much as we're taking care of ourselves by helping ourselves." Several of the responses reject financial ability as the determining factor for receiving healthcare citing—"Money should not be the reason that some people get healthcare and others do not. It is a necessity, regardless of one's financial situation." A smaller set of responses took a conditional or privilege-based approach suggesting that healthcare is earned or tied to financial means. The idea that healthcare is something individuals must earn, akin to other privileges sharing that "You earn it, you get it." Then a more pragmatic approach offered that improved healthcare is associated with one's ability to pay for better services, "improved healthcare is with money to pay for it." Many responses argue that healthcare should be a universal necessity, not determined by wealth or seen as a privilege for select groups. Others acknowledge the current system's dependency on financial means, even if they don't fully support it. Looking at collective good versus individual responsibility, the responses reflect a tension between viewing healthcare as a societal obligation versus an individual achievement or entitlement. A good number of the responses predominantly reject the notion of healthcare as a privilege, favoring accessibility and fairness (27 "against"; 28 "for"). However, there's an undercurrent of realism about the connection between money and healthcare quality, which complicates the debate. These perspectives put a mirror up to the face of societal discussions about balancing ideals with economic and structural constraints. These responses do reflect the ongoing conflict in healthcare today; is it affordable and should everyone have affordable healthcare (McAdams-Jones and Sharp 2026)?

## What Should Healthcare Professionals Do?

So, what should we health professionals do? Several things noted here would be helpful. We should educate ourselves about skin types as well as cultural types. Education is anecdotal to mitigating ignorance which could perpetuate biases. Providing best practices in healthcare demand we think outside of the general education framework and think more inclusively about people for whom we care who may respond differently by no fault of their own.

## References


Cole, P. D., Hatef, D. A., Taylor, S., & Bullocks, J. M. (2009). *Skin care in ethnic populations.* https://pmc.ncbi.nlm.nih.gov/articles/PMC2884920/pdf/sps23168.pdf

DiStefano, S. (2025, January 17). *Nursing named most trusted profession for 23rd consecutive year.* Johns Hopkins University On the Pulse. https://nursing.jhu.edu/magazine/articles/2025/01/nursing-named-most-trusted-profession-for-23rd-consecutive-year/

McAdams-Jones, D., & Sharp, L. (2026). *Are the tenets of eugenics affecting social learning which shapes our social norms*? https://journals.sagepub.com/doi/10.1177/21582440261420503

United States Department of Health and Human Services. (n.d.-a). *Healthy People 2030: Social determinants of health.* https://odphp.health.gov/healthypeople/priority-areas/social-determinants-health

United States Department of Health and Human Services. (n.d.-b). *Healthy People 2030: Enrollment in higher education.* https://odphp.health.gov/healthypeople/priority-areas/social-determinants-health/literature-summaries/enrollment-higher-education

| Objective<br><br>Upon completion of this lesson, the student will | Content/ Teacher Approach | Learner Activity | Evaluation | AACN Essentials Mapping (AACN, 2026) |
|---|---|---|---|---|
| Identify two common disease presentations or skin abnormalities (such as erythema, cyanosis, jaundice, and infection) on light and dark skin | Explain the physiological role of melanin and its impact on wound healing, pigmentation changes, and disease presentation across diverse skin tones | Divide into groups of four: Group discussions of current understanding of skin physiology | Report out | **Domain 1: Knowledge for Nursing Practice**<br>*1.2a Apply or employ knowledge from nursing science as well as the natural, physical, and social sciences to build an understanding of the human experience and nursing practice*<br>**Domain 2: Person-Centered Care**<br>*2.3c Perform a clinically relevant, holistic health assessment*<br>**Domain 3: Population Health**<br>*3.1 Manage population health*<br>✅ **Rationale:**<br>This objective emphasizes foundational clinical knowledge and recognition of disease presentations. It also integrates awareness of **variation in clinical signs across diverse populations**, directly supporting equitable assessment and reducing diagnostic bias |

| Objective<br>Upon completion of this lesson, the student will | Content/ Teacher Approach | Learner Activity | Evaluation | AACN Essentials Mapping (AACN, 2026) |
|---|---|---|---|---|
| Discuss how different skin abnormalities manifest on light versus dark skin tones | Demonstrate accurate assessment techniques for detecting erythema, cyanosis, jaundice, and infection signs on patients with light and dark skin tones using evidence-based strategies (e.g., palpation, mucous membrane inspection) | Students in groups of two return demonstration to each other | Faculty observe each group | **Domain 2: Person-Centered Care**<br>*2.1b Demonstrate compassionate care*<br>*2.2d Demonstrate the ability to conduct sensitive or difficult conversations*<br>*2.2f Demonstrate emotional intelligence in communications*<br>*2.3c Perform a clinically relevant, holistic health assessment*<br>**Domain 3: Population Health**<br>*3.1h Describe general principles and practices for the clinical management of populations across the age continuum*<br>*3.1i Identify ethical principles to protect the health and safety of populations being served*<br>**Domain 9: Professionalism**<br>*9.1a Apply principles of professional nursing ethics and human rights in patient care and professional Situations*<br>*9.1b Reflect on one's actions and their consequences*<br>*9.1c Demonstrate ethical behaviors in practice*<br>✅ **Rationale:**<br>This objective moves beyond recognition into **critical thinking and discussion of disparities**. It aligns strongly with your expertise in **health equity and SDOH**, emphasizing culturally responsive care and addressing systemic gaps in clinical training |

| Objective<br><br>Upon completion of this lesson, the student will | Content/ Teacher Approach | Learner Activity | Evaluation | AACN Essentials Mapping (AACN, 2026) |
|---|---|---|---|---|
| Apply appropriate assessment techniques to ensure equitable and accurate clinical evaluation on light and dark skin | Discuss the value of cultural humility and equity in clinical practice by recognizing how implicit bias and systemic factors affect diagnosis and treatment in patients with different skin tones | Pair students and give an opportunity to express their value systems relative to caring for patients of different skin color | Offer the groups an opportunity to share their value systems prior this lesson and compare to their value systems post this lesson | **Domain 2: Person-Centered Care**<br>*2.3c Perform a clinically relevant, holistic health assessment*<br>*2.4a Synthesize assessment data in the context of the individual's current preferences, situation, and experience*<br>**Domain 3:Population Health**<br>*3.1g Participate in the implementation of sociocultural and linguistically responsive interventions*<br>**Domain 6: Interprofessional Partnerships**<br>*6.1e Communicate individual information in a professional, accurate, and timely manner*<br>**Domain 9: Professionalism**<br>*9.1a Apply principles of professional nursing ethics and human rights in patient care and professional situations*<br>*9.1b Reflect on one's actions and their consequences*<br>*9.1c Demonstrate ethical behaviors in practice*<br>✅ **Rationale:**<br>This objective reflects **application-level learning** (higher-order Bloom's), directly tied to **safe, equitable clinical practice**. It supports AACN's emphasis on:<br>• Eliminating bias in assessment<br>• Ensuring diagnostic accuracy across diverse populations<br>• Using evidence-based strategies |

## References

American Association of Colleges of Nursing. (2026). *The essentials: Core competencies for professional nursing education.* https://www.aacnnursing.org/Portals/0/PDFs/Publications/Essentials-2026.pdf

Cole, P. D., Hatef, D. A., Taylor, S., & Bullocks, J. M. (n.d.) *Skin care in ethnic populations.* https://pmc.ncbi.nlm.nih.gov/articles/PMC2884920/pdf/sps23168.pdf

DiStefano, S. (2025, January 17). *Nursing named most trusted profession for 23rd consecutive year.* Johns Hopkins University On the Pulse. https://nursing.jhu.edu/magazine/articles/2025/01/nursing-named-most-trusted-profession-for-23rd-consecutive-year/

McAdams-Jones, D., & Sharp, L. (2026). *Are the tenets of eugenics affecting social learning which shapes our social norms*? https://journals.sagepub.com/doi/10.1177/21582440261420503

United States Department of Health and Human Services. (n.d.-a). *Healthy People 2030: Social determinants of health.* https://odphp.health.gov/healthypeople/priority-areas/social-determinants-health

United States Department of Health and Human Services. (n.d.-b). *Healthy People 2030: Enrollment in higher education.* https://odphp.health.gov/healthypeople/priority-areas/social-determinants-health/literature-summaries/enrollment-higher-education

II

# Healthcare as a Right or a Privilege

## LESSON OBJECTIVES

Upon completion of this lesson, the student will:

a. Analyze the ethical, legal, and economic arguments that support healthcare as a human right versus a social privilege, using evidence from at least three scholarly or policy sources.
b. Evaluate how different healthcare models (e.g., U.S. system vs. universal healthcare systems) reflect the "right versus privilege" debate and compare their impact on health outcomes and equity.
c. Apply concepts of social determinants of health to explain how the classification of healthcare as a right or a privilege affects vulnerable populations and contributes to health disparities.

## INTRODUCTION

In America, healthcare is available but not always accessible. This is generally because healthcare for all intents and practical purposes has become a commodity that is bought and sold; it is not free. So, when did healthcare become commodified? We can look at ourselves as healthcare providers aiming every second to provide the most effective care in the most efficient and cost-saving manner while operating under a tight budget that limits time with the patient as well as limits resources. The two dynamics are at odds. Healthcare is viewed in terms of cost versus profit often before the patient (Lenzer, n.d.). The question being pushed by some healthcare providers comes from the altruistic point of view regarding healthcare as a right leaning on the system of reform to provide care for everyone. There is still the more pragmatic view that raises the conversation of cost and who will bear the cost of resources for those recipients who cannot pay. A troubling conundrum indeed.

## HEALTHCARE AS A RIGHT VERSUS A PRIVILEGE

When looking at U.S. healthcare from a compassionate perspective, we see selfless commentary by way of providers; healthcare is a right. When looking at healthcare from a cost perspective, we see frugality amid possible waste with a huge concern that healthcare is a privilege accessible to only those who can pay for it. But then, even others would argue, healthcare is essential to life, to our dignity, and to societal well-being, which would make it a human right. The further the disconcerting opinions deeply resonate, the further the divide and the wider the disparity gap. Research has supported that better and more available healthcare improves society by improving outcomes and reducing long-term cost (Heineman & Froemke, 2013; Rudiger, 2008). Furthermore, Dr. Don Berwick, in the documentary Escape Fire (Heinman & Froemke, 2013), advocates for unencumbered access for all using the best available science that supports better outcomes. In looking at statistics, the United States is not number #1 in chronic healthcare management (Heineman & Froemke, 2013). If the path to healthcare is decided by payment, and it is decided by payment in the United States, then those living without healthcare insurance or the means to pay for healthcare will likely suffer the most. From this point of reference, it can be understood how healthcare became a commodity.

There are reasons for looking forward with a plan for universal healthcare. Jones and Kantarjian (2015) note that many European countries have had some degree of universal healthcare for centuries. Much of the lean into this model was to preserve the economy by avoiding loss of wages due to illness and to stabilize income of the general working population. Also, these countries subscribe to the idea that healthcare is a basic human right. The United States, South Korea, Mexico, and Turkey are the only countries that do not subscribe to the thinking that healthcare is a human right; thus, the consumer must pay for their healthcare (Jones & Kantarjian, 2015).

## STRUCTURAL INEQUITIES

*Structural inequities and access to essential resources.* It is a fact that healthcare is core to social determinants of health because alone, and by itself as a singular factor, it can influence a person's income level through available employment types and whether or not a person is able to complete an educational program. Furthermore, the neighborhood where a person lives can decide if those persons are able to access healthcare due to availability or lack of availability. This availability is explained through understanding city planning, for example, where healthcare facilities are placed in relationship to different neighborhoods. Racial compositions of neighborhoods tend to be mostly homogenous with the lower-income population residing in a different part of the town than those persons who belong to the higher-income category. Incomes are also ultimately a dividing force on the level of economy where race becomes more synonymous with lower incomes than higher incomes (Hanewald, Berthold and Stingl, 2023). Research consistently shows that individuals of lower socioeconomic status experience worse health outcomes and their life expectancy is reduced due to reduced access to timely, affordable medical care. Papadimos (2007) emphasizes that more than 45 million Americans were uninsured or underinsured, with poverty, race, occupation, and education being major structural obstacles to obtaining needed care. When healthcare is framed as a privilege, these inequities deepen because the ability to not only access but also to pay for healthcare becomes the gateway to survival rather than a shared societal obligation.

### Inequitable Access Perpetuates Disparities in Healthcare Outcomes

Pushing a sentiment of "healthcare as a right" against the view that "healthcare is a privilege" frames how systems respond to disparities produced by social determinants of health (SDoH). Al Mojil (2025) argues that when healthcare is recognized as an "inviolable human right," policies become oriented toward eliminating financial barriers, expanding Medicaid, and ensuring preventive care—interventions proven to reduce population-level disparities.

Contrariwise, managing healthcare as a privilege underpins market-based access, leaving individuals defenseless to shattering health and financial outcomes, as noted by Jones and Kantarjian (2015), who cite common U.S. experiences of losing homes, savings, or even access to life-saving treatments due to inability to pay. Here is produced a circular loop where structural disadvantage—poverty, racial discrimination, housing instability—translates into defeated healthcare outcomes, less-than-desirable disease outcomes, and higher mortality. These facts shine the light on a singular healthcare model versus a universal healthcare model. In a universal healthcare model, the principles are more centered on the right to healthcare in opposition to a multiple-payer healthcare model that leaves gaps between who has a right and who is privileged to access and receive healthcare. Remember, healthcare begins in the community, not in the hospitals.

## HUMAN RIGHTS

Health policy can more purposely address SDoH when healthcare is addressed as a right by expanding coverage, financially supporting community health programs, and promoting early intervention systems. Maruthappu et al. (2013) illustrate how reforms such as the Affordable Care Act move U.S. healthcare closer to universalism by reducing the uninsured population and reframing care as a social obligation. International human rights frameworks are adamant with this approach as they link dignity, equality, and social stability directly to health—informing us how closely aligned the principles are with population-level SDoH strategies. If healthcare is viewed as a privilege, this will give society permission to normalize unequal health outcomes as expected or deserved, but, when viewed as a right, it is illuminated that health inequities reflect policy failures rather than individual shortcomings. Educating society is essential for creating just, equitable healthcare systems that respond to societies experiencing the effects of social determinants shaping health.

### Why Is This Important

Fundamental to the science of healthcare, it is a fact that nutrition, rest, exercise, and regular preventive care are key components to create and maintain a healthy body while regulating hormones, avoiding inflammation, and ultimately supporting brain function. When the body is in a homeostatic condition of communication and response, the brain receives the oxygen, nutrients, and energy it needs to think clearly, mitigate stress, preserve emotional stability, and make healthy decisions. Chronic pain associated with physical illness conversely can increase anxiety, alter a mood, and force more difficulty when surviving daily tasks. Thus, it could be argued that a healthy mind is dependent upon a healthy body and a healthy body is dependent upon a healthy mind. Both are heavily influenced by tenets of social determinants of health.

## What Should Healthcare Professionals Do?

As healthcare professionals, it is imperative that we can: advocate for equitable access at the point of entry to healthcare; in a multiplayer system, those patients with insurance or those who can afford to pay for their healthcare often experience a smoother and faster transition through the health system. Alternately, without insurance and a means to pay for healthcare, patients are more likely to experience delays and maybe even less-than-adequate care. We can intervene with healthcare managers, social workers, and community resources in advocating for equitable and timely care. Remember, care delayed is care denied.

Next, because as healthcare professionals we are one of the most trusted voices for the public, we can use our voices to influence health policy, by speaking to Congress, speaking at hearings on healthcare affordability, educating the public, speaking out in the community, educating other healthcare workers and joining in full support of medicine and other healthcare professional organizations.

Finally, we strive always to provide culturally safe and bias-free healthcare while supporting colleagues similarly. In a multiplayer system, bias can easily creep in to discriminate against the patient without insurance or underinsured or without funds to purchase care. Healthcare providers are key to mitigating this imbalance by ensuring all patients receive high-quality care that is timely, unbiased with accessible accommodations thereby providing trauma-informed and dignity-centered practices. Lastly, as healthcare professionals, we should always be involved in organizational policy championing for community partnerships and tracking for disparities in outcomes by payer status using some method such as an equity dashboard.

## References

Al Mojil, F. (2025). *Access to healthcare in the United States: A fundamental right or a privilege? Journal of Student Research, 14*(1). https://doi.org/10.47611/jsrhs.v14i1.8450

Buckley, T. (2024, March 9). *Healthcare: Right, privilege or neither. Brownstone Institute.* https://brownstone.org/articles/health-care-right-privilege-or-neither/

Hanewald, B., Berthold, D., & Stingl, M. (2023). *Does the human right to healthcare apply universally? A contribution from a trauma therapeutic perspective. International Journal of Environmental Research and Public Health, 20*(15), 6492. https://doi.org/10.3390/ijerph20156492

Heineman, M., & Froemke, S. (2013). *Escape fire: The race to save America's healthcare* [DVD].

Jones, G. H., & Kantarjian, H. (2015). *Health care in the United States—Basic human right or entitlement? Annals of Oncology, 26*(10), 2193–2195. https://doi.org/10.1093/annonc/mdv321

Lenzer, J. (n.d.). *Money talks: Profit before patients.*

Maruthappu, M., Ologunde, R., & Gunarajasingam, A. (2013). Is health care a right? Health reforms in the USA and their impact upon the concept of care. *Annals of Medicine and Surgery, 2*(1), 15–17. https://doi.org/10.1016/S2049-0801(13)70021-9

Papadimos, T. J. (2007). Healthcare access as a right, not a privilege: A construct of Western thought. *Philosophy, Ethics, and Humanities in Medicine, 2*, Article 2. https://doi.org/10.1186/1747-5341-2-2

Rudiger, A. (2008). From market competition to solidarity? Assessing the prospects of U.S. health care reform plans from a human rights perspective. *Health and Human Rights, 10*(1), 123–135. https://doi.org/10.2307/20460089

| Objective<br>Upon completion of this lesson, the student will | Content/Teacher Approach | Learner Activity | Evaluation | AACN Essentials Mapping (AACN, 2026) |
|---|---|---|---|---|
| Analyze the ethical, legal, and economic arguments that support healthcare as a human right versus a social privilege, using evidence from at least three scholarly or policy sources | Provide articles on:<br>Affordable Healthcare Act<br>Human rights<br>Moral duty to ensure healthcare access<br>Discuss in class | Read the following articles:<br>**Maruthappu et al. (2013)**—Discusses the Affordable Care Act, disparities in access, and the moral question of whether healthcare is a right or entitlement<br>**Al Mojil (2025)**—Argues that healthcare is an "inviolable human right" supported by economic benefits, workforce productivity, and constitutional principles<br>**Papadimos (2007)**—Uses major Western philosophers (Kant, Rawls, Hobbes, Paine, Arendt) to argue that societies have a moral duty to ensure healthcare access | Complete a **one-page evidence summary** that identifies:<br>One ethical argument supporting healthcare as a right<br>One legal argument<br>One economic argument<br>One counterargument supporting healthcare as a privilege<br>Students must cite all three sources in their summary | **Domain 1**<br>**Knowledge for Nursing Practice**<br>*1.2c: Demonstrate social responsibility as a global citizen who fosters the attainment of access to healthcare for all*<br>*1.2d: Examine influence of personal values in decision-making for nursing practice*<br>*1.2e Demonstrate ethical decision-making*<br>✅ ***Rationale:***<br>This objective helps students analyze economic and structural barriers to healthcare access and gives support to foster equal access to healthcare for all |

| Objective<br>Upon completion of this lesson, the student will | Content/Teacher Approach | Learner Activity | Evaluation | AACN Essentials Mapping (AACN, 2026) |
|---|---|---|---|---|
| Evaluate how different healthcare models (e.g., U.S. system vs. universal healthcare systems) reflect the "right versus privilege" debate and compare their impact on health outcomes and equity | Discuss patients accessing and navigating different health systems across the globe | Pre-class preparation readings (individual work)<br>Wagner, E., & Cox, C. (2025, October). *International comparison of health systems* https://www.kff.org/global-health-policy/health-policy-101-international-comparison-of-health-systems/?entry=table-of-contents-introduction<br>The Common Wealth Fund. (2024). *Mirror, mirror 2024: A portrait of the failing U.S. health system: Comparing performance in 10 nations.* https://www.commonwealthfund.org/publications/fund-reports/2024/sep/mirror-mirror-2024<br>Debate pros and cons of 10 global healthcare systems compared to the U.S. healthcare system | Develop a 10-minute simulation-based scenario (use any format) that includes a patient navigating one of the healthcare systems from access point to discharge point<br>Discuss in class | **Domain 3 Population Health**<br>*3.1e: Apply an understanding of the public health system and its interfaces with clinical healthcare in addressing population health needs*<br>*3.1: Assess population health data*<br>**Domain 6**<br>**Interprofessional Partnerships**<br>*6.3a: Integrate the roles and responsibilities of healthcare professionals through interprofessional collaborative practice*<br>**Domain 9 Professionalism**<br>*9.6c: Integrate core principles of collective well-being and human rights into practice*<br>✅ ***Rationale***<br>This objective prepares students to critically evaluate systems and advocate for change |

| Objective<br>Upon completion of this lesson, the student will | Content/Teacher Approach | Learner Activity | Evaluation | AACN Essentials mapping (AACN, 2026) |
|---|---|---|---|---|
| Apply concepts of social determinants of health to explain how the classification of healthcare as a right or as a privilege affects vulnerable populations and contributes to health disparities | Discussion<br>SDoH:<br>>Food<br>>Housing<br>>Transportation<br>>Health insurance<br>>Income | In groups of four analyze and strategize for the following patients (hint: social and community resources)<br>*Patient:* 58-year-old African American mother of two with Type 2 diabetes; works two part-time jobs with no benefits<br>*SDOH factors:* Low income, lacks insurance, food insecurity, barriers to transportation<br>*Impact:* She delays insulin refills due to cost, unable to access specialty care resulting in diabetic foot infection<br>**Evidence link for pre-class readings:** U.S. patients frequently face financial barriers due to voluntary private insurance and gaps in coverage—millions remain uninsured and cost is a leading barrier to care. [kff.org] | 20 minutes for each group for each scenario:<br>Discuss strategies<br>Discuss planned outcomes<br>Discuss patient education<br>Discuss sustainability<br>Discuss how the right-versus-privilege debate affects this case<br>Discuss ethics of care<br>Compare both systems: pros and cons | **Domain 1 Knowledge for Nursing Practice**<br>*1.1b: Apply knowledge of nursing science that develops a foundation for nursing practice*<br>*1.2a: Apply or employ knowledge from nursing science as well as the natural, physical, and social sciences to build an understanding of the human experience and nursing practice*<br>*1.2e: Demonstrate ethical decision-making*<br>*1.3b: Integrate nursing knowledge (theories, multiple ways of knowing, evidence) and knowledge from other disciplines and inquiry to inform clinical judgment*<br>**Domain 2 Person-Centered Care**<br>*2.1a Demonstrate qualities of empathy*<br>*2.1b: Demonstrate compassionate care* |

| Objective<br>Upon completion of this lesson, the student will | Content/Teacher Approach | Learner Activity | Evaluation | AACN Essentials mapping (AACN, 2026) |
|---|---|---|---|---|
| | | *Patient:* 50-year-old woman in Canada with identical health profile.<br>*SDOH factors:* Same socioeconomic challenges (low income, food insecurity), but **guaranteed access** to primary care, essential medications, and follow-up.<br>*Impact:* Receives early intervention, has routine diabetes monitoring, fewer complications, and stable health<br>**Evidence link for preclass readings:** Universal coverage systems (Australia, U.K., Canada, Netherlands) ensure basic healthcare needs are met and achieve better outcomes and equity than the United States, where the system underperforms on access and equity measures (commonwealthfund.org; also ncafcc.org) | | *2.1c: Establish mutual respect with the individual and family*<br>*2.2a: Demonstrate relationship-centered care*<br>*2.2b: Consider individual beliefs, values, and personalized information in communications*<br>*2.2d: Demonstrate the ability to conduct sensitive or difficult conversations*<br>*2.2f: Demonstrate emotional intelligence in communications*<br>**Domain 3 Population Health**<br>*3.1b: Assess population health data*<br>*3.1d: Compare and contrast local regional, national, and global benchmarks to identify health patterns across populations*<br>*3.4a: Describe policy development processes*<br>✓ **Rationale**<br>This objective prepares the student to see real-world consequences of healthcare inaccessibility |

## References

American Association of Colleges of Nursing. (2026). *The essentials: Core competencies for nursing education.* https://www.aacnnursing.org/Portals/0/PDFs/Publications/Essentials-2026.pdf

Kaiser Family Foundation. (n.d.). *KFF polling.* https://www.kff.org/

The Common Wealth Fund. (2024). *Mirror, mirror 2024: A portrait of the failing U.S. health system: Comparing performance in 10 nations.* https://www.commonwealthfund.org/publications/fund-reports/2024/sep/mirror-mirror-2024

Wagner, E., & Cox, C. (2025, October). *International comparison of health systems.* Kaiser Family Foundation. https://www.kff.org/global-health-policy/health-policy-101-international-comparison-of-health-systems/?entry=table-of-contents-introduction

III

# The Controversy: People Who Cannot Contribute to Their Healthcare (Uninsured or Underinsured) Should or Should Not Receive Healthcare

## LESSON OBJECTIVES

Upon completion of this lesson, the student will:

a. Explain how social determinants of health and social risk factors shape patients' ability to access, afford, and engage in healthcare.
b. Apply a contextual, trauma-informed nursing framework when planning care for patients experiencing social risk factors.
c. Demonstrate nursing advocacy by identifying realistic, equity-focused care strategies that preserve patient dignity.

## INTRODUCTION

Having healthcare insurance does not guarantee healthcare. Many areas, particularly rural areas, are known to offer minimal and less-than-optimal healthcare offerings. According to the Institute of Medicine (U.S.) Committee on Monitoring Access to Personal Health Care Services,

> *Access* is a shorthand term for a broad set of concerns that center on the degree to which individuals and groups are able to obtain needed services from the medical care system. Often because of difficulties in defining and measuring the concept, people equate access with insurance coverage or with having enough doctors and hospitals in the geographic area in which they live. But having insurance or nearby healthcare providers is no guarantee that people who need services will get them. Conversely, many who lack coverage or live in areas that appear to have shortages of healthcare resources do, indeed, receive services. (1993)

So, how has this definition further enlightened what is really being said? Can those people who access the care have an opportunity for a good healthcare outcome? In the case where a good outcome can be expected yet it is systemically denied to some certain populations, then there is, in fact, an access concern. Of note, these systemic denials are often not color-coded; lack of access often does not discriminate within those populations experiencing a legacy of poverty. Poverty and healthcare access seem to run parallel to each other. According to the US Department of Health and Human Services, n.d., Healthy People 2030 findings note that a lack of funds or a lack of healthcare insurance can force a person to delay seeking healthcare. Furthermore, even if healthcare is accessed, the reality of the difficulty with paying the bills acquired as a result of the healthcare visit pushes the potential patient to not seek access to healthcare. Healthy People 2030 continued with studies that emphasized the uninsured or underinsured when reaching the age of Medicare or being awarded Medicaid were only then receiving care that diagnosed their chronic illness for which they began to receive treatment.

Access becomes a problem, again, when insurances such as Medicare and Medicaid are not accepted by some physicians. In areas heavily populated with people using Medicare and Medicaid serviced by fewer physicians accepting those insurances produces an access barrier. The problem with lack of or inconvenient transportation can figure into the equation as well. Healthy People 2030 (US Department of Health and Human Services, n.d.) cited the COVID years where racial/ethnic minorities who were more prone to contracting COVID also lacked reliable transportation and lived in areas where healthcare was least available forcing them to travel for healthcare access. Thus, the research is showing that affordability and cost are the biggest reasons the lower socioeconomic class, the uninsured, and the underinsured are delaying and often not seeking healthcare.

## RISK FACTORS OR SOCIAL DETERMINANTS OF HEALTH

Nguyen and Cole (2025) noted that the higher the number of risk factors, the lower the proportion of low socioeconomic population who will seek healthcare. Social risk factors (SRF) are significant and include such things as housing instability, food insecurity, less-than-optimal educational facilities, less-than-optimal community structures, lack of employment, and, ultimately, limited to no access to healthcare, all factors mirroring social determinants of health. Nguyen and Cole (2005) concluded that

> Among 90,208 low-income adults, 46.6 percent reported at least one SRF. Compared to people who reported no SRFs, those who reported four or more were more likely to report being unable to afford care (28.21 percentage points [PP], $p < 0.001$) and less likely to have a personal doctor (−4.98 PP, $p < 0.001$) or routine checkup in the last 2 years (−4.29 PP, $p < 0.001$). The magnitude of disparity by number of SRFs in inability to afford care was larger among privately insured and uninsured people to those with Medicare or Medicaid coverage (Nguyen and Cole, 2005).

Financial barriers are a key to healthcare access, regardless of if it is available or not; money becomes a pivotal factor in decisions concerning whether to purchase insurance, to purchase healthcare, or to even spend any money at all to seek care, as a result of not having a job. Job insecurity can be added as a risk factor and another social determinant of health. Thus, cost of health is a barrier, and research has shown that lower-educated populations versus higher-educated populations largely exist in the lack of affordability populations. This barrier would agree with the findings of Liu and Wadhera (2025) who tagged the United States as facing a healthcare affordability crisis. All of the aforementioned barriers plus those of disparaged and poverty-consumed areas mostly experience and express this affordability crisis. Ultimately, their inability to contribute to their own healthcare is deeply entrenched in social determinants of health (Liu & Wadhera, 2025).

### WHY IS THIS IMPORTANT?

So why is any of this important? This is important because it is possible to mischaracterize people based on their ability to pay for healthcare. Also, personal perceptions about a type of people can cause healthcare providers to allow bias to interfere with their ability to implement best practices in the care of patients. Furthermore, a healthcare provider's thinking about those who can afford to contribute to their healthcare versus those who cannot contribute might possibly direct how a healthcare provider cares for a patient. At a western university, a number of healthcare hopefuls were queried if those who could contribute to their care versus those who could not contribute to their care should receive healthcare. A qualitative design was used with a survey developed and critiqued by expert faculty from nursing; no survey was currently in existence. No psychometrics were performed; thus, this is a survey and not a research tool. Purposive sampling was used selected by a university Institutional Research Team providing emails for nurses and science majors. A Qualtrics survey was distributed. Data were collected and coded and themed. The Institutional Review Board cleared the study.

The questions asked, relative to healthcare, if the participant believed people who do not contribute to their own welfare and the good of our country should or should not benefit from the hard work of others.

> Just under 50% answered in the affirmative that people who do not contribute to their own welfare and the good of our country should not benefit from the hard work of others; the remaining respondents disagreed that people who do not contribute to their own welfare and the good of the country should not benefit from the hard work of others. Fifteen respondents went further to expound on the question. Among those respondents who chose to expound on the question by sharing their thoughts further, eight respondents shared that if they (the person) are not able to work, by default of health or other reasons, then they should receive help. Four respondents shared that if they are able to work, they should work; if they chose not to work then they should not receive help. Two respondents shared that people must work and one respondent shared that all "situations are different and it would depend on the situation." Admittedly, this question was a precursor to "getting at" personal beliefs about the "humanness" in people or the humanity of people; what is the core belief of one human being towards another and if human beings believe they should care for another. It leads into healthcare as a privilege or a right. Those fifteen who expounded had a clear consensus on the observation that this is not a "black or white" situation and that if anything, there should be differentiation on "willing to contribute/work" and "not willing to contribute/work." The opinions as to what extent of the assistance, be it gov-

> ernment or private, was split and overall, the gist was underlying tension between compassion for those who are vulnerable to frustration with what is perceived as abuses in the welfare system. (McAdams-Jones & Sharp, 2026)

This is important because as a healthcare professional, we need to be aware that our thoughts about people affect how we approach them to provide care. As caregivers, our patients trust us to provide for their best interests. In that vein, we should understand and appreciate that how we think can help us become more educated about how we practice.

## What Should Healthcare Professionals Do?

As healthcare professionals, we should be forever learners; we must stay abreast of healthcare and how it is informed by the communities that we serve. We must remember social determinants of health; we must study the phenomenon very carefully so that we understand its context and intent. It is from this place we must practice providing healthcare and caring in the very sense of the words describing social determinants of health. Furthermore, we can educate ourselves about trauma-informed care and how to apply some of its approaches. Trauma-informed approaches connect to the patient's "lasting adverse effects of experiencing traumatic events" (Substance Abuse and Mental Health Services Administration [SAMHSA], 2026, para. 1). Some fundamental principles of trauma-informed care are safety, peer support, trustworthiness and transparency, and collaboration and mutuality with empowerment and voice and choice (SAMHSA, 2026, para. 1). Then, finally, healthcare is situated, not individualized: People are in situations often not of their own individual planning but of their own given situations about which we must constantly remind ourselves and fellow healthcare providers.

## References

Liu, M., & Wadhera, R. K. (2025). The United States faces a healthcare affordability crisis. *BMJ, 390*, r1702. https://doi.org/10.1136/bmj.r1702

McAdams-Jones, D., & Sharp, L. (2026). Are the tenets of eugenics affecting social learning which shapes our social norms? *SAGE Open, 16*(1), 1–14. https://doi.org/10.1177/21582440261420503

Nguyen, K. H., & Cole, M. B. (2025). Social risk factors, health insurance coverage, and inequities in access to care. *American Journal of Preventive Medicine, 68*(1), 145–153. https://doi.org/10.1016/j.amepre.2024.09.005

Substance Abuse and Mental Health Services Administration. (2026, February 8). *Trauma-informed approaches and programs.* https://www.samhsa.gov/mental-health/trauma-violence/trauma-informed-approaches-programs

U.S. Department of Health and Human Services, Office of Disease Prevention and Health Promotion. (n.d.). *Healthy People 2030: Access to health services.* https://odphp.health.gov/healthypeople/priority-areas/social-determinants-health/literature-summaries/access-health-services

| Objective<br>Upon completion of this lesson, the student will | Content/Teacher Approach | Learner Activity | Evaluation | AACN Essentials Mapping (AACN, 2026) |
|---|---|---|---|---|
| 1. Explain how social determinants of health and social risk factors shape patients' ability to access, afford, and engage in healthcare | **Lecture**<br>Introduce key concepts: SDOH, social risk versus social need, structural barriers, and ethical nursing responsibilities | Activity 1: Case Study Analysis (Small Groups—20–30 minutes)<br>**Scenario**<br>A 58-year-old patient with diabetes and hypertension presents repeatedly to the emergency department. The patient is labeled "noncompliant," reports difficulty affording medications, works two jobs, and has unstable housing<br>**Groups of 4 Task:**<br>• Identify at least three **social determinants or risk factors** affecting care<br>• Reframe the patient's situation using an SDOH perspective | Develop **realistic nursing care plan** that accounts for constraints<br>Hint: Replace Compliance with Realistic Partnership<br>In SDOH-aware nursing, **the goal is not compliance** but **feasible care**<br>Nurses ask:<br>• *What part of this plan is realistic for your life right now?*<br>• *What gets in the way when you try to care for yourself?*<br>• *What matters most to you today?* | **Domain 3: Population Health**<br>• *Competency 3.1*: Assess population health data<br>• *Competency 3.1c: Assess the priorities of the community and/or the affected clinical populations*<br>**Domain 9: Professionalism**<br>• *Competency 9.3a: Engage in advocacy that promotes the best interest of the individual, community, and procession*<br>• *9.2g: Communicate in a professional manner*<br>• *9.3f: Demonstrate adherence to a culture of civility*<br>✅ **Rationale:**<br>This objective emphasizes foundational understanding of how health engages a community as it drives access to healthcare in the system |

| Objective<br>Upon completion of this lesson, the student will | Content/Teacher Approach | Learner Activity | Evaluation | AACN Essentials Mapping (AACN, 2026) |
|---|---|---|---|---|
| 2. Apply a contextual, trauma-informed nursing framework when planning care for patients experiencing social risk factors | **Lecture**<br>Social determinants of health versus social risk factors<br>Cost, insurance gaps, housing instability, and access barriers<br>Reframing "nonadherence" as constrained choice | Using the same scenario employing guided reflection (15 minutes), in **Groups of Four Task:**<br>1. Examine bias, assumptions, and moral distress<br>2. Discuss ways to mitigate bias, assumptions, and moral distress<br>3. Apply trauma-informed tenets to care of this patient | Reflective Discussion (Individual or Group—15 minutes)<br>Learners respond (written or verbal):<br>How does this patient's context challenge traditional notions of compliance?<br>What assumptions might healthcare providers bring into this encounter?<br>How does nursing ethics guide care when patients cannot contribute financially? | ***Domain 2: Person-Centered Care***<br>• *Competency 2.1: Engage with the individual in establishing a caring relationship*<br>• *Competency 2.2: Communicate effectively with individuals*<br>***Domain 3: Population Health***<br>• *Competency 3.3: Consider the socioeconomic impact of the delivery of healthcare*<br>***Domain 6: Interprofessional Partnerships***<br>• *Competency 6.1: Communicate in a manner that facilitates a partnership approach to quality care delivery*<br>• *Competency 6.4d: Collaborate with interprofessional team members to establish mutual healthcare goals for individuals, communities, or populations*<br>***Domain 9: Professionalism***<br>• *9.1a: Apply principles of professional nursing ethics and human rights in patient care and professional situations* |

| Objective<br>Upon completion of this lesson, the student will | Content/Teacher Approach | Learner Activity | Evaluation | AACN Essentials Mapping (AACN, 2026) |
|---|---|---|---|---|
| | | | | **Rationale:**<br>This objective includes the concept of trauma-informed care addressing multiple social risk factors |
| Demonstrate nursing advocacy by identifying realistic, equity-focused care strategies that preserve patient dignity | Reframing Advocacy in Nursing Practice<br>**Advocacy is not "fixing" the patient** or persuading them to comply with an ideal plan. Advocacy is the intentional use of **power, knowledge, and professional voice** to ensure care is:<br>• **Realistic** within the patient's life circumstances<br>• **Equitable**, not identical<br>• **Dignity-preserving**, not deficit-based<br>Advocacy begins when a nurse recognizes that *the standard plan does not fit the patient's reality* | A 52-year-old patient with heart failure is readmitted for fluid overload. The chart documents "poor compliance with diet and medications." The patient works hourly shifts, has no consistent transportation, and cannot afford all prescriptions. Housing is stable but food access is limited<br>**(20 minutes) Group of Four Task:**<br>Each group will identify **one advocacy-based care strategy** that is: | Written or Verbal:<br>Each group presents:<br>• **One care modification**<br>• **One advocacy action** (bedside or team level)<br>• **One language change** that preserves dignity<br>Hint: Instead of insisting on ideal diet changes, the nurse asks what foods are affordable and accessible | **Domain 9: Professionalism**<br>• *Competency 9.1: Demonstrate an ethical comportment in one's practice reflective of nursing's mission to society*<br>• *Competency 9.1c: Demonstrate ethical behaviors in practice*<br>• *Competency 9.1g: Advocate for the individual's right to self determination*<br>**Rationale:**<br>This objective includes the concept of the patient's rights seated in advocacy of patient equity |

| Objective<br>Upon completion of this lesson, the student will | Content/Teacher Approach | Learner Activity | Evaluation | AACN Essentials Mapping (AACN, 2026) |
|---|---|---|---|---|
| | Micro (Bedside Advocacy)<br>• Identifying cost-related nonadherence<br>• Negotiating achievable care goals<br>• Using respectful, contextual language in documentation<br>Meso (Team/System Advocacy)<br>• Speaking up in rounds when plans are unrealistic<br>• Involving social work or case management early<br>• Questioning discharge plans that set patients up to fail<br>Macro (Professional Advocacy)<br>• Supporting policies that expand access<br>• Educating peers on SDOH<br>• Challenging stigmatizing practices or labels | 1. Realistic<br>2. Equity-focused<br>3. Dignity-preserving | Instead of assuming medication refusal, the nurse explores cost, side effects, work schedules, or housing instability | |

## References

American Association of Colleges of Nurses. (2026). *The essentials: Core competencies for nursing education*. https://www.aacnnursing.org/Portals/0/PDFs/Publications/Essentials-2026.pdf

Nguyen, K. H., & Cole, M. B. (2025). Social risk factors, health insurance coverage, and inequities in access to care. *American Journal of Preventive Medicine, 68*(1), 145–153. https://doi.org/10.1016/j.amepre.2024.09.005

Substance Abuse and Mental Health Services Administration. (2026, February 8). *Trauma-informed approaches and programs.* https://www.samhsa.gov/mental-health/trauma-violence/trauma-informed-approaches-programs

U.S. Department of Health and Human Services, Office of Disease Prevention and Health Promotion. (n.d.). *Healthy People 2030: Access to health services.* https://odphp.health.gov/healthypeople/priority-areas/social-determinants-health/literature-summaries/access-health-services

# IV

# The Concept of Eugenics Situating Health Professions

## LESSON OBJECTIVES

Upon completion of this lesson, the student will:

a. Analyze the historical foundations of eugenics and its integration into healthcare practice
b. Examine how eugenic ideologies contributed to bias, othering, and health disparities in healthcare practice.
c. Apply ethical principles to evaluate and respond to the legacy of eugenics in practice.

## INTRODUCTION

The history of eugenics presents one of the most ethically troubling intersections between science, medicine, and social ideology. Originating in the late 19th century, eugenics was promoted as a scientific means of improving human populations through selective reproduction. However, in practice, it evolved into a system that justified discrimination, exclusion, and coercive medical interventions against marginalized populations. The involvement of healthcare professionals in the advancement and legitimization of eugenics complicates contemporary understandings of professional ethics in medicine and nursing (Pernick, 1997).

McAdams-Jones and Sharp (2026) emphasize that eugenic ideologies did not operate in isolation but were embedded in processes of social learning that shaped norms, attitudes, and behaviors. Their work underscores how historical frameworks of superiority and inferiority continue to influence social and healthcare interactions, often leading to "othering" and inequitable outcomes (McAdams-Jones & Sharp, 2026). Within this context, examining eugenics is essential for situating healthcare professionals as moral agents responsible for upholding ethical standards such as justice, autonomy, and respect for human dignity. This discussion explores the historical context of eugenics, its integration into healthcare practice, and its ethical implications. Furthermore, the discussion will seek to analyze how healthcare professionals can reconcile this legacy by committing to ethical principles and critical reflection in modern practice.

Healthcare professionals—particularly physicians and nurses—played a central role in legitimizing and operationalizing eugenic ideologies. Medicine, as a trusted and authoritative discipline, provided scientific credibility to eugenic claims, even when those claims were based on flawed or incomplete understandings of genetics (Elby, 2025). Physicians were instrumental in advocating for and performing sterilization procedures, often framing these interventions as necessary for public health and societal improvement. Similarly, nurses and public health professionals were involved in educating communities, promoting eugenic ideals, and identifying individuals considered "unfit" for reproduction (Skeen & Wall, 2023).

The integration of eugenics into healthcare was not purely coercive; it was also reinforced through professional education and socialization. Nurses, for instance, were often taught to view eugenics as a means of improving population health and reducing social problems. This professional alignment with eugenic principles highlights the influence of social norms and institutional structures on healthcare practice (Skeen & Wall, 2023).

McAdams-Jones and Sharp (2026) highlight the concept of "social learning" as a mechanism through which such ideologies are transmitted. Healthcare professionals, as members of society, are not immune to these influences. Instead, they may internalize prevailing beliefs about hierarchy, worth, and normalcy, which can shape their interactions with patients. The complicity of healthcare professionals in eugenics reflects a broader ethical dilemma: how individuals within a profession dedicated to healing and care can become agents of harm when guided by flawed social and scientific assumption (Eby, 2025).

## SOCIAL LEARNING, OTHERING, AND HEALTHCARE

A key contribution of McAdams-Jones and Sharp's work (2026) is its focus on the role of social learning in shaping perceptions of others. According to McAdams-Jones and Sharp (2026), Bandura's Social Learning Theory proposes that individuals acquire behaviors, attitudes, and values through observation and interaction within their social environment. In the context of eugenics, this means that discriminatory beliefs about race, ability, and worth were learned and reinforced through cultural and institutional practices. The concept of "othering"—viewing certain individuals or groups as fundamentally different or inferior—is central to understanding the persistence of eugenic thinking. McAdams-Jones and Sharp (2026) note that healthcare professionals and patients alike may engage in othering, which can negatively affect patient outcomes.

Historically, othering justified the exclusion of marginalized groups from equitable healthcare and supported interventions such as sterilization or institutionalization. Today, remnants of these attitudes can still be observed in health disparities, implicit bias, and unequal access to care. For example, research has shown that structural hierarchies—rooted in race, class, and ability—continue to influence health outcomes and disparities. These disparities are not merely the result of biological differences but, in fact, are shaped by social determinants of health and systemic inequalities (Lagerwey, 2020). Understanding the role of social learning in perpetuating these patterns is critical for healthcare professionals. It highlights the need for ongoing education, self-reflection, and institutional change to challenge harmful norms and promote equity.

### Why Is This Important

Healthcare professionals are fundamentally guided by ethical principles such as beneficence (acting in the patient's best interest), nonmaleficence (avoiding harm), autonomy (respecting individuals' right to make decisions about their own care), and justice (ensuring fairness and equity in treatment). However, the history of eugenics reveals a profound distortion of these principles, particularly when societal interests were prioritized over the dignity and rights of individuals.

Eugenics, especially in the late 19th and early 20th centuries, was often framed as a scientific and public health strategy intended to "improve" the population. Under this ideology, certain individuals and groups—often those marginalized by disability, poverty, race, immigration status, or perceived "social deviance"—were deemed unfit to reproduce. Healthcare professionals, operating within these systems, played roles in implementing policies such as forced sterilizations and institutionalizations. These actions were justified under the premise of benefiting society, yet they directly violated the ethical obligation to prioritize the well-being and autonomy of individual patients.

The physical harms of these interventions were severe and irreversible, including loss of reproductive capacity and, in some cases, complications or death from procedures. Equally significant were the psychological and social consequences: trauma, stigma, loss of identity, and intergenerational impacts on families and communities. Individuals subjected to sterilization often had no informed consent and were denied the ability to exercise their civil rights. These actions represent clear violations of autonomy and justice, and they underscore how medical authority can be misused when shaped by discriminatory ideologies.

Importantly, the involvement of healthcare professionals ranged along a spectrum. Some knowingly participated in these practices, aligning with prevailing scientific and social beliefs of the time. Others may have been complicit without full awareness, constrained by institutional roles, policies, and power structures. This complexity does not diminish responsibility but rather highlights the importance of ethical vigilance and critical reflection within professional practice.

Understanding this history is essential for modern healthcare professionals. It serves as a cautionary example of how bias—whether explicit or implicit—can influence clinical judgment and decision-making. The legacy of eugenics contributes to mistrust in healthcare systems among affected communities, particularly those historically targeted by these policies. This mistrust can impact healthcare utilization, patient–provider relationships, and health outcomes.

The connection to Social Determinants of Health (SDOH) is especially significant. Many of the inequities observed in present-day health outcomes—such as disparities in access to care, education, housing, and economic opportunity—are rooted in historical practices of exclusion, discrimination, and othering. Eugenics-based policies reinforced social hierarchies and contributed to the marginalization of entire populations, effects that persist across generations.

## What Should Health Professionals Do?

Understanding the history of eugenics places a responsibility on modern healthcare professionals to actively prevent similar ethical failures. When ethical principles are challenged, clinicians must move beyond passive awareness to intentional, equity-centered action. We must validate patients' values, cultural perspectives, and lived experiences in decision-making. We should question policies and practices that obviously or even appear to disproportionately harm certain groups. In doing so, we should continue to engage in ethics education and case review. We must critically think and judge our actions and actions of other healthcare professionals when a decision seems to be for "societal good" but is at the expense of an individual or group; this poses an ethical danger zone.

These are the times to speak up, participate in ethics committees and policy committees, and become the patients' advocate through advocacy organizations. Furthermore, recognize that current disparities are rooted in historical injustices, which are stemming from societal ills such as eugenics. Ensure that screening for housing, food insecurity, and access to healthcare are included in the interview and initial encounter. Know the resources available to the patients and the community and ensure the two are connected. Acknowledge historical harms openly and honestly when appropriate. Practice transparency in communication and shared decision-making. Support culturally safe and trauma-informed care models.

## References

Eby, M. R. (2025). Expertise and the "new science" of eugenics. *Social Science & Medicine, 369*, 117829. https://doi.org/10.1016/j.socscimed.2025.117829

Lagerwey, M. D. (2020). Eugenics and healthy families. *Ethics in Natural and Human Environment, 3(1).* https://doi.org/10.25974/enhe2020-3en

McAdams-Jones, D., & Sharp, L. (2026). Are the tenets of eugenics affecting social learning which shape our social norms? *SAGE Open, 16*(1), 1–14. https://doi.org/10.1177/21582440261420503

Pernick, M. S. (1997). Eugenics and public health in American history. *American Journal of Public Health, 87*(11), 1767–1772. https://doi.org/10.2105/AJPH.87.11.1767

Skeen, K., & Wall, B. M. (2023). Nursing and eugenics in the early 20th century United States. *Nursing Outlook, 71*(5), 102018. https://doi.org/10.1016/j.outlook.2023.102018

| Objective<br>Upon completion of this lesson, the student will | Content/Teacher Approach | Learner Activity | Evaluation | AACN Essentials Mapping (AACN, 2026) |
|---|---|---|---|---|
| 1. Analyze the historical foundations of eugenics and its integration into health-care practice | A. Introduction to Eugenics<br>• Definition of eugenics: a movement aimed at "improving" the human population through con-trolled reproduction<br>• Origins in the late 19th century (Francis Galton).<br>• Connection to emerging fields: genetics, public health, and social reform<br>B. Social and Scientific Context<br>• Influence of Social Dar-winism and misinterpre-tation of natural selection<br>• Role of industrialization, immigration concerns, and class structures<br>• How "fitness" was socially constructed (disability, poverty, race, etc.)<br>C. Eugenics in Healthcare Practice<br>• Role of healthcare professionals: | In groups of two, create a visual timeline of key events in eugenics history and healthcare involvement | Share the visual timelines and discuss how the healthcare involvement affected patient outcomes, then and now | 1. **Domain 1** Examine how eu-genic ideologies contributed to bias, othering, and health dis-parities in healthcare practice<br>**Knowledge for Nursing Practice**<br>*1.2a :Apply or employ knowledge from nursing science as well as the natural, physical, and social sci-ences to build an understanding of the human experience and nursing practice*<br>*1.2c: Demonstrate social respon-sibility as a global citizen who fosters the attainment of access to healthcare for all*<br>*1.2d:Examine influence of person-al values in decision-making for nursing practice*<br>*1.2e:Demonstrate ethical decision-making*<br>**Domain 2 Person-Centered Care**<br>*2.1a: Demonstrate qualities of empathy* |

| Objective<br>Upon completion of this lesson, the student will | Content/Teacher Approach | Learner Activity | Evaluation | AACN Essentials Mapping (AACN, 2026) |
|---|---|---|---|---|
| | ○ Physicians performing sterilizations<br>○ Nurses enforcing institutional policies<br>○ Public health officials promoting population control programs<br>• Forced sterilization laws (e.g., Buck v. Bell, 1927)<br>• Institutionalization of individuals labeled "unfit"<br>• Marriage restrictions and reproductive control | | | *2.1b: Demonstrate compassionate care*<br>*2.1c: Establish mutual respect with the individual and family*<br>*2.2b: Consider individual beliefs, values, and personalized information in communications*<br>✅ **Rationale:** This objective exposes how scientific ideas can be shaped by social, political, and cultural contexts. Eugenics connects to major historical events such as immigration policies, healthcare betterment, racial segregation, and the Holocaust. It demonstrates how scientific ideas can be misapplied to justify inequality and harm. It provides essential lessons about ethics, respect for diversity, and the importance of safeguarding human rights in science and society |

| Objective<br>Upon completion of this lesson, the student will | Content/Teacher Approach | Learner Activity | Evaluation | AACN Essentials Mapping (AACN, 2026) |
|---|---|---|---|---|
| 2. Examine how eugenic ideologies contributed to bias, othering, and health disparities in healthcare practice | A. Ideology<br>• Belief in improving populations through selective reproduction<br>• Constructing bias: implicit and explicit attitudes influencing judgment<br>• Othering: process of labeling certain groups as different, inferior, or less worthy<br>• Health disparities: preventable differences in health outcomes among populations<br>B. Flawed Science<br>• Use of pseudoscience to justify hierarchy (race, disability, class)<br>• Medical labeling (e.g., "feebleminded," "unfit")<br>• Assumptions about worth, productivity, and social value<br>• Role of diagnostic criteria shaped by social norms | In groups of four, research one of the concepts (ideology, flawed science, division of people or resulting harm) and give at least two examples of how the concept affected healthcare access and outcomes during eugenics and post-eugenics | Present your findings with the class (30 minutes) using any technology deemed suitable to convey research | **Domain 3**<br>**Population Health**<br>*3.1b: Assess population health data*<br>*3.1c: Assess the priorities of the community and/or the affected clinical population*<br>*3.1e: Apply an understanding of the public health system and its interfaces with clinical healthcare in addressing population health needs*<br>*3.1g: Participate in the implementation of sociocultural and linguistically responsive interventions*<br>*3.1h: Describe general principles and practices for the clinical management of populations across the age continuum*<br>*3.1i: Identify ethical principles to protect the health and safety of populations being served* |

| Objective<br>Upon completion of this lesson, the student will | Content/Teacher Approach | Learner Activity | Evaluation | AACN Essentials Mapping (AACN, 2026) |
|---|---|---|---|---|
| | C. Creating Division of People<br>• Construction of “desirable” vs. “undesirable” populations<br>• Religions: Christianity vs. labeling non-Christians<br>• Segregation in institutions and care delivery<br>• Dehumanization in clinical decision-making<br>• Language in medical records reinforcing stigma<br>D. Resulting Harm<br>• Limited access to care for targeted groups<br>• Forced sterilization and reproductive injustice<br>• Unequal resource allocation (institutional vs. community care)<br>• Long-term intergenerational health and socioeconomic effects | | | ☑ **Rationale:** This objective provides understanding that bias in healthcare is not accidental—it has **historical roots in ideologies like eugenics**, which ranked human worth based on perceived biological <u>traits.</u> It equips learners with the critical, ethical, and clinical awareness needed to provide **equitable, culturally responsive, and justice-oriented care** |

| Objective<br>Upon completion of this lesson, the student will | Content/Teacher Approach | Learner Activity | Evaluation | AACN Essentials Mapping (AACN, 2026) |
|---|---|---|---|---|
| 3. Apply ethical principles to evaluate and respond to the legacy of eugenics in practice | Core ethical principles<br>• **Autonomy**: Respecting individuals' rights to make informed decisions about their care<br>• **Beneficence**: Acting in the best interest of the patient<br>• **Nonmaleficence**: Avoiding harm<br>• **Justice**: Ensuring fairness and equity in care | Class discussion identifying each principle with an example of how that principle was realized or not realized in healthcare, past and present | Class participation | *3.4b: Describe the impact of policies on population outcomes, including access to healthcare resources for populations being served*<br>*3.4d: Propose modifications to or development of policy based on population findings*<br>*6.4a: Demonstrate an awareness of one's biases and how they may affect mutual respect and communication with team members*<br>*6.4c: Engage in constructive communication to facilitate conflict management*<br>*7.3d: Recognize internal and external system processes and structures that perpetuate practices that contribute to lack of opportunities or access and any other form of treatment that is based on differences within healthcare*<br>*9.1e: Report unethical behaviors when observed* |

| Objective<br>Upon completion of this lesson, the student will | Content/Teacher Approach | Learner Activity | Evaluation | AACN Essentials Mapping (AACN, 2026) |
|---|---|---|---|---|
| | | | | **Domain 10 Personal, Professional, and Leadership Development**<br>*10.3g: Demonstrate self-awareness of one's own biases and their relationship to one's culture and environment*<br>✅ **Rationale:** This objective constructs advanced, action-oriented understanding that goes beyond knowledge into ethical and professional behavior leading to ethical decision-making. Furthermore, it helps the student to critically examine the lasting effects of eugenics and take informed, responsible action. It prepares them to practice with integrity, equity, and a commitment to protecting human dignity |

## References

American Association of Colleges of Nursing. (2026). *The essentials: Core competencies for nursing education.* https://www.aacnnursing.org/Portals/0/PDFs/Publications/Essentials-2026.pdf

Eby, M. R. (2025). Expertise and the "new science" of eugenics. *Social Science & Medicine, 369,* 117829. https://doi.org/10.1016/j.socscimed.2025.117829

Lagerwey, M. D. (2020). Eugenics and healthy families. *Ethics in Natural and Human Environment, 3(1).* https://doi.org/10.25974/enhe2020-3en

McAdams-Jones, D., & Sharp, L. (2026). Are the tenets of eugenics affecting social learning which shape our social norms? *SAGE Open, 16*(1), 1–14. https://doi.org/10.1177/21582440261420503

Pernick, M. S. (1997). Eugenics and public health in American history. *American Journal of Public Health, 87*(11), 1767–1772. https://doi.org/10.2105/AJPH.87.11.1767

Skeen, K., & Wall, B. M. (2023). Nursing and eugenics in the early 20th century United States. *Nursing Outlook, 71*(5), 102018. https://doi.org/10.1016/j.outlook.2023.102018

# V

# Supporting the Health of Others Who May Not Look Like Me

## LESSON OBJECTIVES

Upon completion of this lesson, the student will:

a. Increase self-awareness and reflective practice
b. Develop cultural humility through active learning
c. Apply inclusive and respectful care strategies in practice

## INTRODUCTION

In healthcare, we often enter practice believing that our clinical knowledge, past experiences, and beliefs about our world immersed in our good intentions are enough to provide effective care. Yet, as we encounter patients whose lives, approaches to living, identities, cultures, and lived experiences differ from our own, we often realize that **competence alone does not guarantee understanding**. Supporting the health of people who do not look and approach life like us, live like us, or experience the world as we do requires something more intentional.

We could argue that it is very difficult to talk about a subject if we do not have knowledge of it. Then, we also know that we do not often challenge our beliefs; our beliefs about things and people in the world are at best based on our experiences before our education, and neither they are all-encompassing. For the many, many, subjects about people, their appearances, their culture, if we admitted the truth to ourselves, most of us would agree we need more education about the lives of others. Yet, in our busy lives, those things are not as important as getting through the challenges of just existing in our daily circle or orbit. Thus, it is realized from a professional standpoint, the work begins with **looking inward before reaching outward**. Each of us brings our own background, beliefs, and assumptions into the care environment—shaped by culture, education, privilege, hardship, and lived experience. These perspectives influence how we interpret patients' behaviors, their approaches to life, their decisions, which all ultimately affect their health outcomes. To care equitably, we must first learn to recognize how our own lived experiences and beliefs shape what we see, shape our biases—and fuel those things that we may overlook.

## PANNING THE VIEW

At the same time, ethical, accurate, culturally competent, and effective care demands that we **step beyond ourselves**. This means reading books such as this one (which is merely a start, but a healthy start); listening to patients as experts in their own lives; seeking to understand the social, cultural, and structural forces that shape their health; and resisting the urge to rely on assumptions or stereotypes. This means asking yourself, "How can I learn more versus condemning yourself or the system because you realize you are ill-equipped to competently manage this clinical space?" Learning about others is not a one-time achievement; it is a continuous practice of curiosity, humility, and relationship-building.

In this space, our goal is not to master every culture or experience. Rather, it is to develop the capacity to ask better questions, to remain open when discomfort arises, and to respond in humility with care that honors dignity, difference, and shared humanity. Furthermore, our goals should be to learn about the subjects that impact our work, namely, people. If we were electrical engineers servicing a product with different codes and standards than our customary codes and standards, we would research for understanding as the consequences from not knowing could be lethal. Similarly, as nurses, we are often given "new and improved" equipment that will require us to be in-serviced. Often the in-servicing is on the spot with another nurse; yet we are in-serviced in some way. This is necessary to prevent misuse of the product/equipment that could cause harm to the patient or even to the nurse versus the intended or desired improvement of care. In sum, we should periodically in-service ourselves about the different people in our community as these same people may come to us for care. The American Nurses Association's Position Statement on *The Nurse's Role and Responsibility in Unveiling and Dismantling Systems of Oppression: Protecting and Promoting Inclusive Strategies in Practice Settings, Policy, and Advocacy* asks us to recognize our position in a system that oppresses some people and to

1. Call on nurses and their allies to learn about, reflect on, and, most importantly, act to end oppression in all its forms. 2. Identify how nursing is situated within and as part of systems of oppression that function as organized systems, structures, and practices that harm patients, foster health inequity, perpetuate injustice, constrain nurses, and instigate social violence. 3. Support nursing and nurses' ability to recognize their role in upholding or uprooting practices that harm patients, foster health inequity, perpetuate injustice, and instigate social violence. 4. Articulate the complexities of discrimination as a function of systems of oppression, as well as nursing strategies toward ending all forms of discrimination that construct, reinforce, or amplify oppression, violence, and inequity. (2025)

We also see barriers to care when the language is different. Although healthcare has made strides in conquering language barriers, Panayiotou et al. (2019) note that there are many translation apps available; however, the professional interpreter remains the gold standard. We must communicate accurately and effectively with our patients in spite of the fact that it would be so much easier if we all spoke the same language. When providers commit to reflection, learning, and inclusive practice, advocacy becomes possible—not as an abstract ideal, but as a daily expression of respect, equity, and professional responsibility.

As we move forward with this lesson, we will explore how self-awareness, cultural humility, and intentional advocacy allow us to support the health of individuals and communities different from ourselves—and how this effort strengthens not only patient outcomes but also our integrity as healthcare professionals.

## Why Is This Important

We learn from those who teach us. Hoffman et al. (2016) note that healthcare has suffered a long history of erroneous, pseudoscientific, and flawed science explaining pain tolerance in people. Instead of teaching culturally informed approaches for pain assessment, the training in health professions (medicine, para professions, nursing) relative to pain has been inadequate in challenging racialized myths rooted in 19th-century ideations that melanated skin is thicker, has less sensitive nerve endings, or a higher pain tolerance (Hoffman et al., 2016). The narrative went further to note how the darker-skinned (melanated) patients received less-than-optimal care management and were rated lower in the need for care relative to the non-melanated patients. Essentially, erroneous education has translated into suboptimal and negligent care (Hoffman et al., 2016). We are reminded of Dr. J. Marion Sims' lack of concern for the physical or emotional health of slave women in denying them anesthesia during experimental surgeries (Vaswani et al., 2024). These citations are a few of the many that have reported how academics misled its scholars and practitioners causing severe distress, pain, and possibly harm to those under their care. We must lead out with the truth, reminding ourselves and coaching our colleagues through moving away from what we know to be false and erroneous science. Without the truth in healthcare, we make mistakes. Mistakes can be harmful and they can also be lethal.

## What Should Health Professionals Do?

This is our clarion call to reach out beyond ourselves and learn about those around us and those from other cultures. We do live in a global society, and, with transportation being open to the world, we cannot deny that our interactions with people from continents other than ours will continue. Sociology Institute (2025) noted that the impact of globalization is most visible in our daily lives as we see the degree of cultural mixing attributed to not just people but also music, food, and media along with goods across borders bringing us values, enriching societies and hopefully bringing with-it, cross-cultural understanding (2025, para. 5). By failing to correct false biological narratives and by excluding cultural humility from pain education, language and customs education, folkways and mores in education, and providing resources for students to reach outside themselves and learn, healthcare educators have not only misinformed learners but have also institutionalized inequity. Correcting these disparaging practices requires strong repudiation of "color of skin" myths. We have to, post haste, integrate sociocultural frameworks into all aspects of healthcare teaching and learning. We must be accountable as health professionals and educate our upcoming providers in preventing ongoing, avoidable suffering.

## References

Hoffman, K. M., Trawalter, S., Axt, J. R., & Oliver, M. N. (2016). Racial bias in pain assessment and treatment recommendations, and false beliefs about biological differences between Blacks and Whites. *Proceedings of the National Academy of Sciences of the United States of America, 113*(16), 4296–4301. https://doi.org/10.1073/pnas.1516047113

Panayiotou, A., Gardner, A., Williams, S., Zucchi, E., Mascitti-Meuter, M., Goh, A. M., You, E., Chong, T. W., Logiudice, D., Lin, X., Haralambous, B., & Batchelor, F. (2019). Language translation apps in health care settings: Expert opinion. *JMIR mHealth and uHealth, 7*(4), e11316. https://doi.org/10.2196/11316

Sociology Institute. (2025, October 11). *The multidimensional effects of globalization in society.* https://sociology.institute/economic-sociology/effects-globalization-society-multidimensional/

The American Nurses Association. (2025). *The nurse's role and responsibility in unveiling and dismantling systems of oppression: Protecting and promoting inclusive strategies in practice settings, policy, and advocacy (Position statement).* https://www.nursingworld.org/globalassets/practiceandpolicy/nursing-excellence/ana-position-statements/unveiling-and-dismantling-systems-of-oppression_final_bodapproved.pdf

Vaswani, H. K., Kshirsagar, S., Kathpalia, S., & Denge, A. (2024). A pioneer in women's health, Dr. James Marion Sims (1813–1883). *Cureus, 16*(11), e74733. https://doi.org/10.7759/cureus.74733

| Objective<br>Upon completion of this lesson, the student will | Content/Teacher Approach | Learner Activity | Evaluation | AACN Essentials Mapping (AACN, 2026) |
|---|---|---|---|---|
| Practice self-awareness and reflective practice | **Lecture with class discussion**<br>a. Patient perspective on diversity-sensitive care encompasses multiple components, from patient-centered care to concordant care<br>b. Exploring practitioners' uncertainty; emotional responses and continued education | **In groups of four, conduct a 20-minute Discussion:** How we as healthcare providers critically examine our own identities, assumptions, and lived experiences and how these influence interactions with patients from different racial, cultural, social, or economic backgrounds, recognizing that self-awareness is foundational to equitable care | Create a quick-fact educational pamphlet/brochure designed for practitioners that<br>a. Discusses key points in providing culturally sensitive care<br>a. Highlights barriers and pitfalls to avoid in providing culturally sensitive care<br>Selected Articles: Lauwers, et.al., 2024. Marjadi, et.al., 2023, Vandecasteele, et.al., 2024. Swierad & Huang, 2021. You may use other articles as well. | ***Domain 1***: *Knowledge for Practice*<br>*1.2d: Examine the influence of personal values in decision-making for nursing practice*<br><br>***Domain 9*: *Professionalism***<br>*9.1a: Apply principles of professional nursing ethics and human rights in patient care and professional situations*<br>*9.1b: Reflect on one's actions and their consequences*<br>*9.1c: Demonstrate ethical behaviors in practice*<br>*9.1d: Change behavior based on self and situational awareness*<br>✅ **Rationale:** This objective helps to shape the student into safe, reflective, and patient-centered nurses |

| Objective<br>Upon completion of this lesson, the student will | Content/Teacher Approach | Learner Activity | Evaluation | AACN Essentials Mapping (AACN, 2026) |
|---|---|---|---|---|
| Develop cultural humility through active learning | **Lecture with class discussion**<br>a. The value in seeking knowledge about the lived experiences, values, and health challenges of individuals and communities different from self<br>b. The value of engaging in ongoing learning, listening, and relationship-building rather than relying on assumptions or stereotypes | **Class Positionality Reflection: 3 minutes in silence**<br>This is a thought activity: NO sharing required but is allowed if offered<br>Who am I in relation to social determinants of health…to my moral compass?<br>Where did I start (womb) and what is my assessment of where I am and where I intend to go? | Positionality Reflection (10–15 minutes) NO SHARING required but if desired sharing will be accepted<br>Students respond in writing to 3–4 prompts:<br>>What identities do I bring into professional or learning spaces?<br>>When have my assumptions shaped how I interpreted another person's behavior?<br>>What makes me uncomfortable when I think about "getting it wrong"? | ***Domain 2*** *Person-Centered Care*<br>*2.2d: Demonstrate the ability to conduct sensitive or difficult conversations*<br>*2.2e:Use evidence-based patient teaching materials, considering health literacy, vision, hearing, social awareness, and adaptability*<br>*2.2f:Demonstrate emotional intelligence in communications*<br>✅ **Rationale:** This objective trains the student to provide more personalized, patient-centered care instead of relying on stereotypes or assumptions |

| Objective<br>Upon completion of this lesson, the student will | Content/Teacher Approach | Learner Activity | Evaluation | AACN Essentials mapping (AACN, 2026) |
|---|---|---|---|---|
| Apply inclusive and respectful care strategies in practice | Lecture and class discussion<br>a. The effects of social determinants of health and their reflection in society<br>b. How social determinants of health affect healthcare outcomes<br>c. Integrating culturally responsive, dignity-preserving approaches into clinical decision-making<br>d. Willingness vs. ability to seek healthcare | In groups of 4, discuss<br>**Scenario A: Language and Health Literacy** A patient with limited English proficiency nods during discharge teaching but does not ask questions and later demonstrates misunderstanding of medication instructions<br>**Scenario B: Identity and Respect** A patient reports feeling dismissed after staff repeatedly used incorrect terminology to describe the patient's family structure or personal identity<br>**Scenario C: Socioeconomic Barriers** A patient is labeled "noncompliant" because follow-up appointments were missed, but transportation and work schedules were never discussed | After discussion:<br>Each group presents to the class participants their solution/plan to make the patient's visit more inclusive and respectful. Include:<br>1. Inclusive and respectful behaviors that did not happen<br>2. How these inclusive and respectful behaviors could better have been incorporated into the visit<br>Selected articles: Swierad & Huang, 2021, LaVeist & Pierre, 2014, Vrtikapa, Hoque & Hoque, 2025. You may use other articles as well | *Domain 2: Person-Centered Care*<br>*2.1a: Demonstrate qualities of empathy*<br>*2.1b: Demonstrate compassionate care*<br>*2.1c: Establish mutual respect with the individual and family*<br>*2.2a: Demonstrate relationship-centered care*<br>*2.2b: Consider individual beliefs, values, and personalized information in communications*<br>*2.2c: Use a variety of communication modes appropriate for the context*<br>*2.2d: Demonstrate the ability to conduct sensitive or difficult conversations* |

| Objective<br>Upon completion of this lesson, the student will | Content/Teacher Approach | Learner Activity | Evaluation | AACN Essentials mapping (AACN, 2026) |
|---|---|---|---|---|
| | | **Scenario D: Disability and Access** A patient with a mobility or sensory impairment reports difficulty accessing care spaces and feeling rushed during visits | | *2.2e: Use evidence-based patient teaching materials, considering health literacy, vision, hearing, social awareness, and adaptability*<br>*2.2f: Demonstrate emotional intelligence in communications*<br>✅ **Rationale**: This objective prepares the student not just for clinical competence; it also teaches them to be inclusive, respectful, and patient-centered in every interaction. |

## References

American Association of Colleges of Nursing. (2026). *The Essentials: Core competencies for nursing education.* https://www.aacnnursing.org/Portals/0/PDFs/Publications/Essentials-2026.pdf

Lauwers, E. D. L., Vandecasteele, R., McMahon, M., De Maesschalck, S., & Willems, S. (2024). The patient perspective on diversity-sensitive care: A systematic review. *International Journal for Equity in Health, 23*(1), 117. https://doi.org/10.1186/s12939-024-02189-1

LaVeist, T. A., & Pierre, G. (2014). Integrating the 3Ds—Social determinants, health disparities, and health-care workforce diversity. *Public Health Reports, 129*(Suppl. 2), 9–14. https://doi.org/10.1177/00333549141291S204

Marjadi, B., Flavel, J., Baker, K., Glenister, K., Morns, M., Triantafyllou, M., Strauss, P., Wolff, B., Procter, A. M., Mengesha, Z., Walsberger, S., Qiao, X., & Gardiner, P. A. (2023). Twelve tips for inclusive practice in healthcare settings. *International Journal of Environmental Research and Public Health, 20*(5), 4657. https://doi.org/10.3390/ijerph20054657

Swierad, E. M., & Huang, T. T. (2021). It starts with a conversation: The importance of values as building blocks of engagement strategies in community-centered public health research. *International Journal of Environmental Research and Public Health, 18*(6), 2940. https://doi.org/10.3390/ijerph18062940

Vandecasteele, R., Robijn, L., Willems, S., De Maesschalck, S., & Stevens, P. A. J. (2024). Barriers and facilitators to culturally sensitive care in general practice: A reflexive thematic analysis. *BMC Primary Care, 25*(1), 381. https://doi.org/10.1186/s12875-024-02630-y

Vrtikapa, K., Hoque Urmy, F., & Hoque, F. (2025). Social determinants of health: The impact of this overlooked vital sign. *Journal of Brown Hospital Medicine, 4*(3), 138072. https://doi.org/10.56305/001c.138072

# VI

# Division Shaped by Social Norms: Eugenic Legacies, Healthcare Access, and Social Learning

## LESSON OBJECTIVES

Upon completion of this lesson, the student will:

a. Define eugenics and explain its historical origins and principles.
b. Analyze the impact of eugenics on healthcare policy and social norms.
c. Apply Social Learning Theory to understand how societal attitudes toward people, health, and privilege evolve.

## INTRODUCTION

The idea of eugenics was widely embraced in the early 20th century across Europe and the United States, influencing policies such as forced sterilization, restrictive immigration laws, and institutionalization. As health professionals, we are often expected to explain many things that are a quandary for the patient. The purpose of this lesson is to acquaint the reader with an understanding of how social norms are driven by many components in society, to include environmental, social, and economical to name a few (Bandura, 1971). One societal component of some years past is the eugenics movement. Eugenics is the practice or advocacy of improving the genetic quality of the human population through controlled, selective reproduction. It speaks to both positive eugenics, which encourages individuals labeled as genetically "desirable" to reproduce, and negative eugenics that forces a halt of reproduction among those critiqued as "unfit"—including through coercive and deceptive measures such as sterilization or prohibition on marriage (Black, 2003). The concept originated in the late 19th century with Sir Francis Galton, influenced by Darwinian evolution, and was widely imposed on American society into the early 20th century—sponsored by academics, policymakers, and implemented in U.S. laws that were shared worldwide. Immigration was hugely affected and eugenicists factored immigrants as undesirable and contributing to negative eugenics. Immigration laws were fueled by eugenics' faulty footing lacking any scientific evidence. Eugenics became discredited after the depression of the 1920s which caused many otherwise well-born to become unemployed, penniless in soup lines changing their value and rendering them less productive and less desirable. Hence, the purest of an explanation for social determinants of health evolved showing America the flawed science of eugenics.

## IMPACT ON HEALTHCARE

Although explicit eugenic policies have largely been discredited due to their association with human rights abuses—most notably in Nazi Germany—the underlying assumptions about genetic "fitness" continue to shape healthcare practices and social norms today, often in more subtle ways. In modern healthcare, one of the most significant areas of influence is genetic screening and reproductive decision-making (National Human Genome Research Institute, n.d.). Technologies such as prenatal testing, carrier screening, and preimplantation genetic diagnosis (PGD) allow prospective parents to identify genetic conditions in embryos or fetuses. While these technologies are often framed as empowering individual choice and preventing suffering, they also echo eugenic logic by implicitly valuing certain lives over others. For example, the widespread screening for conditions like Down syndrome has led to high rates of pregnancy termination in some regions, raising ethical questions about inclusion, disability rights, and societal attitudes toward difference (Dive & Newson, 2022).

Another impact is seen in how healthcare prioritizes prevention and risk reduction. Public health initiatives often emphasize lifestyle choices and genetic predispositions, which can inadvertently reinforce the notion that individuals are responsible for their biological "quality." This can lead to stigmatization of those with chronic illnesses, disabilities, or conditions perceived as preventable, reflecting a residual eugenic mindset that equates health with moral worth. Additionally, disparities in access to advanced medical technologies may create new inequalities, where those with greater resources can exert more control over reproductive outcomes, echoing earlier class-based and racial biases of eugenic movements (Dive & Newson, 2022).

Social norms have also been shaped by these lingering ideas. There remains a cultural emphasis on optimization—of bodies, intelligence, and productivity—which aligns with the eugenic ideal of improvement. This is evident in the popularity of genetic testing services, wellness industries, and even emerging discussions about gene-editing technologies like CRISPR (Gostimskaya, 2022). While these innovations hold promise for treating disease, they also raise concerns about "designer babies" and the possibility of reviving eugenic thinking under a new, more technologically advanced guise.

## HEALTHCARE AND SOCIAL NORMS

Furthermore, implicit biases in healthcare providers and institutions may reflect enduring stereotypes about certain populations. Historical eugenic ideologies often targeted marginalized groups, including people with disabilities, racial minorities, and the poor. Today, these groups may still experience differential treatment, skepticism, or reduced access to care, suggesting that the social hierarchies reinforced by eugenics have not been fully dismantled (Gillman et al., 2024; National Human Genome Research Institute, n.d.). In conclusion, while overt eugenics has been rejected, its core tenets continue to influence healthcare practices and social expectations. The challenge today lies in balancing scientific advancement with ethical responsibility, ensuring that respect for diversity and individual dignity remains central in both medical decision-making and societal values.

Contemporary debates over healthcare and social welfare reveal enduring divisions shaped by historical legacies and the social norms through which individuals and communities learn, internalize, and reproduce attitudes (Bandura, 1971). Whereas classical eugenic positions advocated restricting resources—sometimes including healthcare—to those deemed "unfit," contemporary responses increasingly foreground equity, contextual fairness, and social responsibility beyond genetic determinism (Black, 2003). These shifts, however, are neither uniform nor complete, and they are mediated by social learning processes that shape community-level norms (Bandura, 1971).

Historically, eugenics was closely intertwined with racial classification, promoting hierarchies of "purity" and presumed superiority (Black, 2003). In stark contrast, McAdams-Jones and Sharp 2026 noted that many contemporary respondents of their survey rejected the use of skin color as a basis for categorizing individuals, signaling a critical normative departure from foundational premises of eugenic thought. This movement reflects broader societal commitments to individual dignity and equal regard, even if these commitments remain contested in some quarters. Social Learning Theory (Bandura, 1971) offers a valuable analytic lens for understanding this transition: Individuals acquire beliefs and behaviors through observation, modeling, and reinforcement, and these socially mediated processes can either reproduce entrenched hierarchies or catalyze normative change (Bandura, 1971). The growing data from this study that rejected racial classification and immigration bans can be interpreted as a learned social norm that increasingly prioritizes inclusivity and anti-discriminatory values, shaped by exposure to diverse communities, evolving educational content, and institutional signals.

A related source of division concerns conditionality—whether access to social benefits should depend upon contribution to society. Such views trace genealogical threads to social Darwinist currents historically embedded in eugenic rationales, which valorized prosperity for the "fittest" and normalized exclusion of the "unfit" (Black, 2003; Hofstadter, 1955). Social Learning Theory helps explain the persistence of these ideas: Norms and attitudes are transmitted intergenerationally, often naturalized within communities as "common sense," and reinforced by elite narratives, policy frames, and local practices (Bandura, 1971). At the same time, many respondents of Mcadams-Jones and Sharp, 2026, articulate a more compassionate orientation that acknowledges structural constraints—such as poverty, discrimination, and health limitations (Social Determinants of Health)—shaping individuals' capacities to contribute. This more context-sensitive view reflects a gradual normative recalibration toward solidarity and recognition of the social determinants of health (Marmot, 2010; WHO Commission on Social Determinants of Health, 2008).

## BANNING IMMIGRATION

Historical policy choices further clarify how access and belonging have been policed through exclusionary criteria. Early-20th-century immigration restrictions were exemplified by the Johnson–Reed Act of 1924, which specifically limited immigrants from Asia and set quotas for Eastern and Southern Europeans. It drew upon eugenic and racialized logics to reconfigure the national community and constrain resource allocation (Black, 2003; Ngai, 2004). In a study examining the idea of othering people, McAdams-Jones and Sharp (2026) noted that 50% of the respondents reported that they were strong opponents of an immigrant ban with a smaller percent agreeing they supported an immigration ban. In thinking about the sentiments on banning immigration that are apparent today, these numbers do not quite reflect what is being shared in the news today considering many of the respondents were against an immigration ban, but as of this writing in 2026, immigration deportations may be the manifestation of stronger immigration bans being implemented across the United States. Contemporary debates about healthcare for non-citizens echo these older rationales, raising questions about worthiness, qualification, and entitlement. Respondents in the present context exhibit division: Some maintain that non-contributors should be ineligible for assistance, while others emphasize providing care to individuals whose health status or circumstances limit their ability to contribute. Notably, many acknowledge that factors beyond individual control—including social and economic conditions—shape health and opportunity, and that these constraints should not foreclose access to care. This recognition represents a meaningful attitudinal shift away from eugenics-aligned gatekeeping toward inclusion and public health protection, even as disagreements persist over financing and delivery mechanisms (Marmot, 2010; McAdams-Jones & Sharp, 2026; WHO Commission on Social Determinants of Health, 2008).

The question of whether healthcare is a right remains contested. Global public health norms increasingly treat healthcare as a right, grounded in the ethical commitment to dignity, equity, and the prevention of avoidable suffering (WHO Constitution, 1946/2006; WHO Commission on Social Determinants of Health, 2008). Yet the mechanisms for realizing that right—whether through public financing, mixed models, or targeted subsidies—remain the subject of policy debate and political contestation. From a social learning perspective, this ongoing deliberation underscores how institutional arrangements, educational curricula, and public discourse can shape the evolution of norms toward more inclusive public health practices (Bandura, 1971).

The sociopolitical context, particularly in educational settings, also influences these dynamics. Resistance to teaching the historical context of race—sometimes framed as protecting students from discomfort—can inadvertently perpetuate burdens on racially marginalized groups and limit shared learning opportunities. Such resistance may slow the societal shift toward equitable norms by undermining informed engagement with historical and structural determinants of inequality (Black, 2003; Ngai, 2004). Social learning processes are pivotal here: What communities choose to teach, endorse, or silence becomes formative, even normative, for the next generation's moral intuitions, policy preferences, and civic behavior (Bandura, 1971).

## Why Is This Important

Taken together, the evidence points to an ongoing evolution away from eugenic rationales and toward more compassionate, equity-oriented understandings of health and social welfare. While divisions persist—around contribution, citizenship, and the design of financing systems—the emergent emphasis on rights, contextualized fairness, and individual dignity suggests that social learning is gradually reshaping norms in ways that support more inclusive public health. Crucially, recognizing the role of social determinants of health and the importance of historically informed education may accelerate this normative shift, enabling institutions to align practice with principles of justice and collective well-being (Marmot, 2010; WHO Commission on Social Determinants of Health, 2008). In this respect, the distancing from racial classification and genetic essentialism marks genuine progress, even as continued vigilance and intentional learning are required to consolidate gains and address the remaining gaps between aspiration and practice.

## What Should Healthcare Professionals Do?

As healthcare professionals, we could *center care on compassion and equity* by shifting away from exclusive ideas rooted in eugenics or genetic essentialism and, instead, prioritize fairness, dignity, and respect for every patient, regardless of background or perceived contribution to society. Then we could *make every effort to recognize Social Determinants of Health (SDOH)* with an understanding that health begins in our communities. We must use culturally sensitive language during patient intake/history and ask the hard questions about social lifestyle, for example, housing, food, and comfort. As healthcare workers, we could strive to understand that health outcomes are shaped by factors like housing, education, income, access to healthcare, and access to resources such as food and comfort. When assessing patients, ask these questions about the patient's community living; consider these broader influences and advocate for interventions that address them. More importantly, strive to discharge the patient in a better place than when the patient was admitted. Furthermore, we should *practice historically informed* care. This means educating ourselves as healthcare providers first and then extend that knowledge to all disciplines on our healthcare team! We must all be aware of the historical context of health disparities and systemic inequities and then advocate for resources that would mitigate inequities. This knowledge helps avoid repeating harmful practices, focuses on meeting the patient where they are, and supports culturally sensitive care with better outcomes. Going further, we want to *treat every patient as a person with rights, not just as a case or condition* while clearly documenting the patient's preferences and rights. This will emphasize that we ensure informed consent, respect autonomy, and involve our patient in decision-making. We must keep our patients safe. An important factor in keeping our patients safe is to never stop learning. In that vein, we should not only be lifelong learners, but we must also *engage in continuous learning* since we can only teach what we know. We must remain vigilant and committed to ongoing education about equity, inclusion, and justice in healthcare. This helps bridge the gap between ideals and real-world practice. Finally, we must collaborate for collective well-being. To engage this principle of collaboration we must intently *work with interdisciplinary teams and community resources* to create holistic care plans that reflect principles of justice and fairness. In collaborating, we share knowledge with peers to promote equity.

## References

Bandura, A. (1971). *Social learning theory.* General Learning Press.

Black, E. (2003). *War against the weak: Eugenics and America's campaign to create a master race.* Four Walls Eight Windows.

Dive, L., & Newson, A. J. (2022). Reproductive carrier screening: Responding to the eugenics critique. *Journal of Medical Ethics, 48*(12), 1060–1067. https://doi.org/10.1136/medethics-2021-107643

Gillman, A. S., Pérez-Stable, E. J., & Das, R. (2024). Advancing health disparities science through social epigenomics research. *JAMA Network Open, 7*(7), e2428992. https://doi.org/10.1001/jamanetworkopen.2024.28992

Gostimskaya, I. (2022). CRISPR–Cas9: A history of its discovery and ethical considerations of its use in genome editing. *Biochemistry (Moscow), 87*(8), 777–788. https://doi.org/10.1134/S0006297922080090

Hofstadter, R. (1955). *Social Darwinism in American thought.* Beacon Press.

Marmot, M. (2010). *Fair society, healthy lives: The Marmot review.* The Marmot Review.

McAdams-Jones, D., & Sharp, L. (2026). Are the tenets of eugenics affecting social learning which shape our social norms? *SAGE Open, 16*(1), 1–14. https://doi.org/10.1177/21582440261420503

National Human Genome Research Institute. (n.d.). *Eugenics and scientific racism.* https://www.genome.gov/about-genomics/fact-sheets/Eugenics-and-Scientific-Racism

Ngai, M. M. (2004). *Impossible subjects: Illegal aliens and the making of modern America.* Princeton University Press.

WHO Commission on Social Determinants of Health. (2008). *Closing the gap in a generation: Health equity through action on the social determinants of health.* World Health Organization.

World Health Organization. (2006). *Constitution of the World Health Organization* (45th ed.). World Health Organization. (Original work published 1946)

| Objective:<br>Upon completion of this lesson, the student will | Content/Teacher Approach | Learner Activity | Evaluation | AACN Essentials Mapping (AACN, 2026) |
|---|---|---|---|---|
| Define eugenics and explain its historical origins and principles<br>Analyze the impact of eugenics on healthcare policy and social norms | Historical context of eugenics: Francis Galton; a $20^{th}$-century movement that influenced immigration laws/bans and the Holocaust/Nazi Germany: The journey of Margaret Sanger and birth control efforts<br>Global influence of eugenics on immigration and the continued ethical failures, sterilization laws, and race betterment<br>The journey of Otto Frank | Create a visual map or infographic of eugenics concepts, effect on immigration, historical milestones, and the journey of Margaret Sanger<br>Write a 500-word reflection that explores sterilization laws, race betterment and their impact on society, marginalized communities, then, and today | Submit visual map/ infographic<br>Submit 500-word essay | **Domain 7: *Systems Based Practice***<br>*7.2b: Recognize the impact of differences in healthcare access, quality of care, and social determinants of health on care outcomes*<br>✅ **Rationale:** This objective helps the student to become more ethically grounded and cautious about policies or practices that may harm vulnerable populations. It helps the student to understand that immigration bans are not new or misplaced on human value; they are intentional and have existed for centuries<br>**Domain 7 *Systems-Based Practice***<br>*7.2b: Recognize the impact of differences in healthcare access, quality of care, and social determinants of health on care outcomes* |

| Objective:<br>Upon completion of this lesson, the student will | Content/Teacher Approach | Learner Activity | Evaluation | AACN Essentials Mapping (AACN, 2026) |
|---|---|---|---|---|
| | | | | *7.3d:Recognize internal and external system processes and structures that perpetuate practices that contribute to lack of opportunities or access and any other form of treatment that is based on differences within healthcare*<br>✅ **Rationale:** This objective helps the student become more cautious and critical of policies that affect patient rights |
| Apply Social Learning Theory to understand how societal attitudes toward people, health, and privilege evolve | The shift from exclusion to inclusion and perhaps back to exclusion: immigration laws today in a country built with and populated by immigrants | In self-selected groups: design a poster titled *From Eugenics to Equity: How Social Learning Shapes Healthcare Norms* | In class: Each group presents poster and discusses *how social learning shapes healthcare norms* | **Domain 9: *Professionalism***<br>*9.2a Employ the use of intentional presence to facilitate shared meaning of the experience between nurse and recipient of care*<br>*9.3a Engage in advocacy that promotes the best interest of the individual, community, and profession*<br>*9.1d Change behavior based on self and situational awareness*<br>*9.1g Advocate for the individual's right to self-determination* |

| Objective: Upon completion of this lesson, the student will | Content/Teacher Approach | Learner Activity | Evaluation | AACN Essentials Mapping (AACN, 2026) |
|---|---|---|---|---|
| | | | | **Rationale:** This objective helps the nursing students connect behavior, culture, and healthcare in a practical, insightful way building strong, values-driven nursing identity |

## Reference

American Association of Colleges of Nursing. (2026). *The essentials: Core competencies for nursing education*. https://www.aacnnursing.org/Portals/0/PDFs/Publications/Essentials-2026.pdf

# VII

# For Those Using Simulation in Education

Note to user: This template can be found on the National League for Nurses Simulation Innovation Center web page under Simulation Design Template 2023. However, you may use any of the multiples of Simulation Templates available on Simulation Center webpages.

Simulation Design Template (Revised February 2023)

George Obu

Change: Nursing Students assume roles at 10-minute stage

| | |
|---|---|
| **Date: Today's Date**<br><br>**Discipline:** Nursing<br><br>**Expected Simulation Run Time:**<br>20 minutes each scenario<br><br>**Location: SIM Lab #1**<br><br>**Today's Date:** | **File Name: ISEP Course Assignment**<br>**Student Level:** Staff Nurses at Hospital<br><br>**Debrief and Guided Reflection Time:**<br>Twice the amount of time that the simulation runs.<br><br>**Location for Reflection:** SIM conference Rm #one |

Brief Description of Patient

**Name:** OBU, George **Pronouns: he, him, they**

**Date of Birth: February 8, 1969** **Age: 55 years**

**Sex Assigned at Birth:** male **Gender Identity:** Cisgender

**Sexual Orientation:** LBGTQ **Marital Status:** Married

**Weight**: 181 **Height**: 6′3″

**Racial Group:** African **Language**: isiZulu and English

**Religion**: Bantu (Democratic Republic of the Congo)

**Employment Status:** Employed/Engineer BOEING

**Insurance Status:** Blue Cross Regence **Veteran Status:** NA

**Support Person:** Husband, **Saul** **Support Phone:** 760-989-9898

**Allergies:** None known **Immunizations:** current

**Attending Provider/Team:** Dr. Broomwald A-Team

**Past Medical History: Genital Warts, COVID, R/O Long COVID**

**History of Present Illness: Periods of SOB causing loss of work**

**Social History:** From Nigeria but moved to United States 10 years ago for work with Boeing; partner unemployed but active with patient's care. Lives in the city close to work. Does not smoke, does not use alcohol or recreational drugs. Exercise at the gym three times/per week; tolerates pretty well; nothing strenuous.

**Primary Medical Diagnosis:** Hx COVID x's one; experiencing shortness of breath and inability to work; lost work time due to illness

**Surgeries/Procedures & Dates:** None to date

**As a summary of the problem and scope** of the simulation I propose, in our homogeneous local population, there is minimal heterogeneity among the patient population. On occasions where a patient's gender presentation is in opposition to their gender assignment at birth, or where a patient is melanated (of color), our students require additional learning experiences to enhance their ability to understand and care for these more diverse populations of patients.

**Problem**: Lack of adequate skill sets and knowledge to care for marginalized populations.

**Kolb's Experiential Learning** Theory will ground this simulation-based learning experience where the learner gains concrete knowledge, reflects on that knowledge, conceptualizes the knowledge, and then applies the concepts in a new space (Wijnen-Meijer, Brandhuber, Schneider, & Berberat, 2022).

Psychomotor Skills Required of Participants Prior to Simulation

1. Speech and Hearing; 2. Ambulatory; 3. Full ROM of all extremities; 4. Operate a Stethoscope and equipment standard to a patient room

2. The participants are hospital staff at a local medical center

Cognitive Activities Required of Participants: There are three scenarios

**Prior to Scenario #1 (Outcome 1)**

Watch and discuss on Canvas assignment discussion; follow prompts: How does the face convey meaning? What message does sitting with crossed legs convey? How should we monitor our faces in conversations? What do you want your recipient to see about you? Think about what you can do to improve your body language.

https://youtu.be/06GyVagAXTA

https://youtu.be/Nmp_-JByPaY

https://youtu.be/VAB9cUlGrRo

**These videos will support the participants in understanding, recognizing, and being aware of body language in a way they can relate and manage what could be perceived as poorly received body language.

## JUST PRIOR THE SIMULATION

Present to the group the principles of SDoH: particularly on location, economics, cultures, and folkways of communities. Have each simulation participant discuss communication methods that could work when caring for those populations profoundly affected by SDoH (Healthy People 2030, US Department of Health and Human Services, n.d.).

**This activity will assist the participants to engage in different communication methods that model best practices in approaching people who are not like them.

Have the participants use their electronic devices to research communication strategies when caring for populations not accustomed to Western medicine. Participants discuss different communication strategies and decide on best practices (Afro News, 2021; Majeed, 2005).

***This will help the participants ground their healthcare approaches in grounded healthcare practices germane to specific areas.

Simulation Learning Outcomes

These general outcomes will be shared with the learners.

Simulation Scenario Outcomes (limit to 3 or 4)

1. Model best practices in communication with diverse patient populations
2. Apply appropriate concepts of social determinants of health
3. Demonstrate an understanding of different cultural customs
4. Compile sources that discuss the traditional healing versus Western medicine in the African continent

Faculty Reference

The Healthcare Simulation Standards of Best Practice™

https://www.inacsl.org/healthcare-simulation-standards

## References

Afro News: The Black Media Authority. (2021, March). *Traditional healing vs. Western medicine in the African continent.* https://afro.com/traditional-healing-vs-western-medicine-in-the-african-continent/

Majeed, A. (2005). How Islam changed medicine. *BMJ, 331*(7531), 1486–1487. https://doi.org/10.1136/bmj.331.7531.1486

U.S. Department of Health and Human Services, Office of Disease Prevention and Health Promotion. (n.d.). *Healthy People 2030: Social determinants of health.* https://health.gov/healthypeople/priority-areas/social-determinants-health

Wainwright, S. F., Shepard, K. F., Harman, L. B., & Stephens, J. (2010). Novice and experienced physical therapist clinicians: A comparison of how reflection is used to inform the clinical decision-making process. *Physical Therapy, 90*(1), 75–88. https://doi.org/10.2522/ptj.20090077

Wijnen-Meijer, M., Brandhuber, T., Schneider, A., & Berberat, P. O. (2022). Implementing Kolb´s Experiential Learning Cycle by Linking Real Experience, Case-Based Discussion and Simulation. *Journal of medical education and curricular development, 9,* 23821205221091511. https://doi.org/10.1177/23821205221091511

Setting/Environment

| | |
|---|---|
| ☐ Emergency Department | ☐ ICU |
| ☒ Medical-Surgical Unit | ☐ OR/PACU |
| ☐ Pediatric Unit | ☐ Rehabilitation Unit |
| ☐ Maternity Unit | ☐ Home |
| ☐ Behavioral Health Unit | ☐ Outpatient Clinic |
| | ☒ Other: Nurse's Station and a patient's room |

Equipment/Supplies (choose all that apply to this simulation)

Patient room with standard equipment; bed, chair, computer, headwall. 02. Prongs, overbed table, water pitcher, bedside stand, Nurse's station with desk, chairs, computer

**Simulated Patient/Manikin(s) Needed:** Standard patients, two males, one African descent with accent in bed and gowned, and one white appearing bearded Muslim dressed male sitting at bedside. Four nurses, 1 SW, and 1 Chaplain

**Actors:** Standard patients/trained actors will be used so emotions and body language may be depicted

**Other Props & Moulage:** See native dress above

| **Equipment Attached to Manikin/ Simulated Patient:** | **Equipment Available in Room:** |
|---|---|
| ☒ ID band | ☒ Bedpan/urinal |
| ☐ IV tubing with primary line fluids running at __ mL/hr | ☒ 02 delivery device (type) prongs |
| ☐ Secondary IV line running at __ mL/hr | ☐ Foley kit |
| ☐ IVPB with __ running at mL/hr | ☐ Straight catheter kit |
| ☐ IV pump | ☐ Incentive spirometer |
| ☐ PCA pump | ☐ Fluids |
| ☐ Foley catheter with __mL output | ☐ IV start kit |
| ☒ 02 | ☐ IV tubing |
| ☒ Monitor attached | ☐ IVPB tubing |
| ☐ Other: | ☐ IV pump |
| | ☐ Feeding pump |
| | ☐ Crash cart with airway devices and emergency medications |
| **Other Essential Equipment:** | ☐ Defibrillator/pacer |
| | ☐ Suction |
| **Medications and Fluids:** | ☐ Other: |
| ☐ Oral Meds: | |
| ☐ IV Fluids: | |
| ☐ IVPB: | |
| ☐ IV Push: | |
| ☐ IM or SC: | |

Roles

| | |
|---|---|
| ☒ Nurse 1 Charge Nurse 20+ years' experience non-melanated female | ☐ Observer(s) |
| ☒ Nurse 2 5+ years' experience non-melanated female | ☐ Recorder(s) |
| ☒ Nurse 3 5+ years' experience non-melanated male | ☒ Family member #1 partner white and male appearing wearing Muslim native dress |
| ☒ Nurse 4 newly licensed female non-melanated | ☐ Family member #2 |
| ☐ Provider (physician/advanced practice nurse) | ☒ Clergy |
| ☒ Social worker male Latina/o/x melanated chaplain (prior military) male AA melanated (pharmacist, respiratory therapist, etc.) | ☐ Unlicensed assistive personnel |
| | ☒ Other: 4 RNs 1 Social Worker 1 Chaplain |

a. 1 newly licensed RN of 1 year (female non-melanated/white)
b. 2 with 5+ years of RN experience (one female and one male non-melanated/white American)
c. 1 charge nurse of >20 years' experience (female non-melanated/white American)
d. 1 chaplain with prior military experience (male melanated [African American])
e. 1 Social Worker (male, Latina/o/x) melanated

Guidelines/Information Related to Roles

**Scenario**

1. Nurse with 1 year of experience is fidgeting and pacing at the nurse's station, mumbling something about "two gays and a Muslim." She sits and stares with a disgruntled face mumbling something about "two gays and a Muslim."
2. Non-melanated male nurse with 5+ years' experience sits with the young nurse and inquires if she needs to talk.

Healthcare staff will engage in research about patients and their partner's culture.

**Script:**

Good morning/afternoon everyone and welcome! This simulation-based experience will help us all acclimate to our space here which is somewhat insulated with our majority religion and ethnic culture situating us in mostly a non-melanated (few to any Black or Brown people) or people from other cultures to our space. Today we will care for different ethnic and gendered people. The overall outcomes: Upon completion of this scenario the learner will:

- Model best practices in communication with diverse patient populations
- Apply appropriate concepts of social determinants of health
- Demonstrate an understanding of different cultural customs
- Compile sources that discuss the traditional healing versus Western medicine in the African continent

We plan to enjoy learning about others and add a few extra knowledge feathers to our cap! Our learning space will be a hospital nursing station and a hospital room. As nurses, chaplain, and social worker we will solve a few problems that often play out in the healthcare world—namely, we are faced with patients whom we rarely if ever see. **NOTE: this is a safe space—what goes on here stays here; we learn and apply the learning in our daily practices, but we do not discuss how our colleagues managed in the simulation; that information remains here. We are learning, so we may need more practice, and that is okay. We practice so we can feel comfortable, and we give each other space to learn and feel good about their learning. We treat all behaviors in the simulation setting as real-life situations. We go into character with the patients, and we become as they are; we all are in the scenario. Our patients are actors trained in their roles. They will respond to you as you interact with them; they will ask questions that are relevant to the scenario; they know your roles; speak to them and treat them as you would a patient coming to you for help. You may touch them (following procedure as you would any patient) for necessary care, to include the physical assessment. There will be among you, a charge nurse with 20+ years' experience, 2 staff RNs with 5+ experience, 1 staff RN with less than 1 year of experience, a chaplain, and a Social worker. ***Because we care, we want to learn more about other people, so this will be a first in a series of new learning experiences! Any questions, so far? ............pause................ Having answered those questions, let us move into the scenario space.

**Environment:** This is the nurse's station; a desk, computer, and some chairs. The computers work and they have a patient simulated chart system loaded. You will merely click the history tab on the computer and acquire your patient's history and concerns, read the report, and begin your day. Here are the roles, you may select—let us read the roles and afterwards; ask any questions you might have (Wainright, Shepard, Harman & Stephens, 2022).

**Charge Nurse**: 20+ years' experience, she has been charge nurse for the floor over 13 years; well respected.

**Male and Female 5+** years' experience knows the floor really well, great mentors to new nurses and often charge the floor in the absence of the charge nurse. Experienced and trusted.

**Less than 1 year's experience** nurse; she is not nuanced in decision-making, she is not assertive, she lived in the area all her life and has never been outside of the state; she does not do well with change and might be described as narrow-minded by default.

**Chaplain is** experienced, military background, traveled, and well-liked by staff.

**Social Worker** is competent, resourceful, and meets people easily.

**Questions? Choose your roles** 😊

Here are the outcomes of the scenario: When we complete the scenario it is the hope that you will

1. Model best practices in communication with diverse patient populations
2. Apply appropriate concepts of social determinants of health
3. Demonstrate an understanding of different cultural customs
4. Compile sources that discuss the traditional healing versus Western medicine in the African continent

**Any questions on the outcomes?**

**Please answer these pre-scenario questionnaires (QR code provided)**

1. What is your opinion of immigrants? Can you tell me more?
2. What is your opinion of African immigrants? Can you tell me more?
3. What is your opinion of Muslims? Can you tell me more?
4. What is your opinion of the LGBTQ community? Can you tell me more?
5. How would you define healthcare? A right or a privilege? Can you tell me more?
6. Why should immigrants be allowed to work here in the United States? Why or why not?
7. When should immigrants receive public assistance? How does you answer resonate with the *American Nurses Association Issues Brief: Nursing Beyond Borders: Access to Health Care for Documented and Undocumented Immigrants Living in the US?*
8. What are your thoughts on religions? Are they all welcome here in the United States?
9. When have you ever lived in a foreign country? Have you ever accessed care in a foreign country?
10. Who do you think has the best healthcare in the world?
11. How do you prepare to converse with others who do not speak your language?
12. How do you prepare to converse with others who are not like you?

**Report Students Will Receive Before Simulation**

(Use SBAR format.)

**Time:** 8am

**Person providing report:** report is taken from the computer; pre-recorded

**Situation:**

**George Obu, age 55 years has been diagnosed with "Long COVID" for about a year now. He is a mechanical engineer but has missed a lot of work due to the shortness of breath.**

**Background:** George is from Nigeria, moved to the United States about a decade ago for work. He and his partner, Saul, live in the city and there is one dog. George has been in the hospital once this year for shortness of breath during the spring; his stay was 1 week. He presented to the emergency room last night very short of breath, wheezing almost and room air sats were in the low eighty's. Oxygen was applied, his sats moved to the ninety's and he has been on 2 L since admission. He is on no medications at home and is on no meds since admitted, besides oxygen at 2l/m nasal prongs. His partner is at the bedside.

**Assessment:** VS: 136/80, HR76 Resp 22 Temp 98 Sats 94 percent on 2 L nasal prongs. General systems are negative; lungs are clear aerating all bases—does report increase shortness of breath on exertion. Is out of bed to chair most of day. Does one lap of the halls after each meal.

**Recommendation:**

**Scenario Progression Outline**

**Patient Name:** George Obu **Date of Birth: July 1969**

**Scenario Objectives:** During and upon completion of this scenario the learner will be

1. Mindful of body language (outcomes a and c)
2. Practice active listening when conversation may be uncomfortable.

This supports the learner in modeling best practices of communication; talk less, observe more (outcomes a, b, and c)

Since the learners have had little to no conversation/education on populations other than those populations that look like them, this learning experience may present uncomfortable conversations leading to body language that communicates negatively. The group will be introduced to principles of SDoH (Social Determinants of Health) particularly on location, economics, cultures, and folkways of communities. Have each simulation participant discuss communication methods that could work when caring for those populations profoundly affected by SDoH (Healthy People 2030).

**This activity will assist the participants engage in different communication methods that model best practices in approaching people who are not like them.

**Prework:** View **https://youtu.be/Nmp_-JByPaY** https://youtu.be/VAB9cUlGrRo

https://youtu.be/a6KnPUJPe8w

| Timing (approx.) | Manikin/SP Actions | Expected Interventions | May Use the Following Cues |
|---|---|---|---|
| **0-1 min**<br><br>**Scene: Nurses Station** | **Inexperienced Nurse**: is mumbling about "2 gays and a Muslim."<br><br>**She sits and stares with a disgruntled face for about 3 minutes.**<br><br>**Non-melanated +5-year experience nurse**: "Do we need to talk? Is there something we need to know? Is the patient okay?"<br><br>**Silence ensues** | **Learners should begin by:**<br><br>• **Noticing body language** | **Role member providing cue:**<br><br>**Cue:** |
| **1-5 min** | **Inexperienced nurse:** "Something is 'off' in there because I do not know what I am supposed to say to people who come here and do not live by our standards!!"<br><br>**Non-melanated +5-year experience nurse**: "Probably a lot of us will feel a bit frustrated but let us go on our intranet and see what we can locate as support for us and support for the patients. We can learn about this together."<br><br>**Non-melanted +5-year experience nurse** accesses intranet and begins to read aloud information about the LGBTQ+ persons.<br><br>**Inexperienced nurse** is fidgety and scowling at her coworker while he continues to read aloud. | **Learners are expected to:**<br><br>• **Notice tone**<br>• **Notice body language**<br>• **Notice disparaging connotations directed at patient perhaps due to ignorance**<br>• **Notice need for education and conversation**<br>• **Notice mentoring by +5-year experience nurse** | **Role member providing cue:**<br><br>**Cue:** |

| | | | |
|---|---|---|---|
| **5-10 min** | **Inexperienced nurse**: "I don't really want to read about people who live unrighteously and are not normal."<br><br>**Non-melanated +5 years experience nurse:** "Should we talk about differences first: We should not judge others."<br><br>**Inexperienced nurse:** "Do as you like! I do not think they should be here and certainly do not deserve care!" | **Learners are expected to:**<br>• **Think about disparaging others for whom they care**<br>• **Think about the charge of a nurse to care for all without prejudice**<br>• **Contemplate "how would you react?"** | **Role member providing cue:**<br><br>**Cue:** |

***At this point, the student nurses will assume all these roles going forward

| Timing (approx.) | Manikin/SP Actions | Expected Interventions/ Learners Are Expected to | May Use the Following Cues |
|---|---|---|---|
| **10-15 min**<br>**Scene: Nurses Station**<br>**Muslim partner of the African patient presents to the nurse's station.** | **Muslim partner speaking to nurse with 5 years of experience:** "Is there any way I could talk with the nurse in charge or a social worker?<br>**Nurse with 5+years' experience:** "Sure, I will get the charge nurse." | • **Notice charge nurse's interaction with African patient and Muslim partner** | |
| **15–17 minutes**<br>**Patient's room** | **Charge Nurse to African Patient: "How can I help you?" (looking at African Patient)**<br>**Muslim Partner speaks: "Because of Obu's continued shortness of breath, he has lost workdays/weeks sometimes and we are needing help with food, gas, and paying our utilities."**<br>**Charge Nurse: Oh, I think I might be able to find someone to help you. Do you mind if I get the Social Worker to come in and speak with you? They often have access to many community resources which could be very helpful."**<br>**Muslim Partner looks at African partner and they both nod to each other, "yes." Then the Muslim partner turns to the Charge Nurse: "Yes, we think that might be a good idea. Thank you!"** | • **Notice the skill with which the charge nurse manages conversation**<br>• **Notice how the Muslim partner picks up the conversation from the African partner**<br>• **Reflect on why the Muslim partner took the conversation** | |

| | | | |
|---|---|---|---|
| **17–20 minutes**<br>**Charge Nurse sits at nurses' station with both 5+ year experience nurses and with the inexperienced nurse and spends 10 minutes discussing and teaching about SDoH** | *****Social worker located and briefed by the Charge Nurse and asked to speak with Patient Obu and his partner.**<br><br>**Charge Nurse to colleagues: Let us talk about Social Determinants of Health (SDoH). Charge nurse pulls up the U.S. Department of Health and Human Services' Healthy People 2030 webpage on SDoH and has a 10-minute educational opportunity with staff nurses.** | • **Notice how education on the spot (teachable moments) enhance learning and supports caring for those in our charge—which could be anyone** | |

**Debrief with meaningful learning using Socratic questioning:**

How is everyone feeling?

Based on the responses, lead into the following questions, and **lead into an order that would align with the participants' perceived feelings, emotions, and responses** and, most importantly, being mindful of body language and practicing active listening.

**Debrief Discussions with meaningful learning**

Point out differences between populations, religions, and cultures receiving Western healthcare

1. What is your opinion of immigrants? Can you tell me more?
2. What is your opinion of African immigrants? Can you tell me more?
3. What is your opinion of Muslims? Can you tell me more?
4. What is your opinion of the LGBTQ community? Can you tell me more?
5. How would you define healthcare? A right or a privilege? Can you tell me more?
6. Where should immigrants be allowed to work here in the United States? Why or why not?
7. When should immigrants receive public assistance? How does you answer resonate with the *American Nurses Association Issues Brief: Nursing Beyond Borders: Access to Health Care for Documented and Undocumented Immigrants Living in the US*?
8. What are your thoughts on religions? Are they all welcome here in the United States?
9. When have you ever lived in a foreign country? Have you ever accessed care in a foreign country?
10. Who do you think has the best healthcare in the world?
11. How do you prepare to converse with others who do not speak your language?
12. How do you prepare to converse with others who are not like you?
13. How did you respond to the actors? Why? Were the actors believable?
14. How did you perceive the moulaged face of the inexperienced nurse?
15. If I perceive floundering and/or discomfort I will remain silent till someone speaks. Silence can be very telling communication.

Based on the responses, lead into the following questions **in an order that would align with the participants' perceived feelings, emotions, and responses** and, most importantly, being mindful of body language and practicing active listening.

Point out differences between populations, religions, and cultures receiving Western healthcare

**Required Completion**

Ten percent of each student's grade is applied post completion of the below two surveys. Follow the barcodes provided and thank you!

Survey/questionnaire #1; Please answer these questions again now, to assess your insights gained from this scenario (Bar code display provided).

1. What is your opinion of immigrants? Can you tell me more?
2. What is your opinion of African immigrants? Can you tell me more?
3. What is your opinion of Muslims? Can you tell me more?
4. What is your opinion of the LGBTQ community? Can you tell me more?
5. How would you define healthcare? A right or a privilege? Can you tell me more?
6. Where should immigrants be allowed to work here in the United States? Why or why not?
7. When should immigrants receive public assistance? How does you answer resonate with the *American Nurses Association Issues Brief: Nursing Beyond Borders: Access to Health Care for Documented and Undocumented Immigrants Living in the US*?
8. What are your thoughts on religions? Are they all welcome here in the United States?
9. When have you ever lived in a foreign country? Have you ever accessed care in a foreign country?
10. Who do you think has the best healthcare in the world?
11. How do you prepare to converse with others who do not speak your language?
12. How do you prepare to converse with others who are not like you?
13. How did you respond to the actors? Why? Were the actors believable?
14. How did you perceive the moulaged face of the inexperienced nurse?

If I perceive floundering and/or discomfort I will remain silent till someone speaks. Silence can be very telling communication.

# VIII
# Conclusion

There is much "to do" about skin color, which is a remarkable biological trait that reflects human adaptation to diverse environments. Its primary contribution lies in the role of melanin, which protects against harmful ultraviolet radiation and influences vitamin D synthesis. These variations in pigmentation are evolutionary responses that enabled survival across different climates (Fairbanks, 2015). Appreciating skin color for these contributions means recognizing it as a testament to human resilience and diversity—a natural characteristic that enriches the human experience.

However, skin color has also been burdened by a social construct that distorts its meaning. Historically, societies have attached value judgments to pigmentation, creating hierarchies that fuel discrimination and inequality. This construct has led to systemic racism, health disparities, and cultural divisions, overshadowing the biological significance of skin color. Instead of celebrating its adaptive purpose, the social lens often reduces skin color to a marker of privilege or disadvantage.

Advancing appreciation requires dismantling these harmful constructs and reframing skin color as a symbol of diversity rather than division. Education, inclusive dialogue, and equitable healthcare practices are essential to shift perceptions. Health professionals play a critical role by acknowledging both the biological and social dimensions of skin color—ensuring that care is free from bias and informed by cultural competence.

Ultimately, skin color should be valued for its contributions to human survival and diversity, not as a basis for social stratification. Embracing this perspective fosters respect, equity, and unity in a world enriched by difference.

The ethical transformation of healthcare professions reflects a deliberate effort to move away from harmful ideologies such as eugenics and toward a more just and inclusive model of care. Organizations like the AARC, AACN, AOTA, APTA, ANA, NLN, AMA, and PAEA professions and their leaders are at the forefront of this change, using codes of ethics and position statements to guide professional behavior and institutional priorities.

By emphasizing dignity, equity, diversity, and accountability, these organizations reshape how healthcare is delivered and experienced. They challenge practitioners to not only provide competent care but also to advocate for systemic change and social justice. In doing so, they ensure that healthcare becomes a field that truly serves all individuals—honoring the complexity, diversity, and inherent value of human life.

Healthcare organizations in the United States are undergoing a profound transformation as they confront and address the legacy and ongoing reality of discrimination within the profession. Through formal statements, ethical frameworks, and educational reform initiatives, organizations such as the ones mentioned above are actively reshaping the culture, priorities, and practices of healthcare. Their work represents a deliberate reckoning with racism and inequity and a commitment to building a more just, inclusive healthcare system. By acknowledging historical harms, redefining ethical responsibilities, and promoting diversity and inclusion, these organizations are changing the face of healthcare in meaningful and lasting ways.

# IX

# Key Takeaways

*Healthcare Is Not Apolitical; It Is Tied to Social Justice*

Across these organizations, several common themes emerge that illustrate how they bring change to healthcare professions:

1. *Re-centering Human Dignity*

   All the codes emphasize respect for the inherent worth of every individual. This foundational value directly opposes any ideology that ranks people based on perceived biological or social characteristics.

2. *Advancing Equity and Justice*

   Each organization explicitly addresses disparities in healthcare and calls for action to reduce inequities. This includes advocating for underserved populations, eliminating discriminatory practices, and promoting access to care.

3. *Promoting Diversity and Belonging*

   Diversity is framed as essential to effective healthcare, not as a problem to be managed. This shift represents a profound departure from past ideologies that sought to control or limit human variation.

4. *Strengthening Ethical Accountability*

   By providing clear standards for professional conduct, these organizations hold practitioners accountable for their actions and decisions. Ethical guidelines serve as a framework for navigating complex issues, including new technologies and evolving societal challenges.

5. *Encouraging Lifelong Learning and Reflection*

   Many of these organizations emphasize the importance of ongoing education, cultural competence, and self-awareness. This supports continuous improvement and helps prevent the reemergence of harmful practices.

6. *Moving Forward: Sustaining Change*

   While significant progress has been made, the work of transforming healthcare professions is ongoing. Ethical codes and position statements provide a foundation, but their impact depends on implementation in education, practice, and policy. Healthcare professionals must actively engage with these principles, applying them in daily interactions with patients and colleagues.

7. *Confronting the Reality of Racism in Healthcare: Shifting the Narrative*

   A crucial first step in addressing discrimination is acknowledging its existence and impact. The *American Nurses Association's Racial Reckoning Statement* represents a significant moment of institutional accountability. In this statement, the ANA openly recognizes that racism is not only present in society but also embedded within nursing practice and healthcare systems through disparities in health outcomes, inequitable access to care, and biases in clinical decision-making disproportionately affecting patients from marginalized communities. The factors contribute to higher rates of chronic illness, maternal mortality, and reduced life expectancy.

8. *Ethical Foundations for Change*

    Ethical frameworks play a central role in guiding how healthcare professionals respond to discrimination. The *National League for Nursing's Ethical Principles for Nursing Education* provides a foundation for cultivating ethical awareness and responsibility among future nurses and other healthcare professionals. These principles emphasize respect for human dignity, fairness, integrity, and accountability—values that directly counter discriminatory practices.

## Suggested/Starter Reading List

Fairbanks, D. J. (2015). *Everyone is African: How science explodes the myth of race.* Prometheus Books.

Gould, S. J. (1981). *The mismeasure of man.* W. W. Norton & Company.

Institute of Medicine. (2002). *Unequal treatment: Confronting racial and ethnic disparities in health care.* National Academies Press. https://www.nationalacademies.org/publications/12875

Reeve, W. P. (2015). *Religion of a different color: The Mormon struggle for whiteness.* Oxford University Press.

Skloot, R. (2010). *The immortal life of Henrietta Lacks.* Crown Publishers.

The Possessive Investment in Whiteness: Racialized Social Democracy and the "White" Problem in American Studies Author(s): George Lipsitz Source: *American Quarterly, Vol. 47*, No. 3 (Sep., 1995), pp. 369-387 Published by: The Johns Hopkins University Press Stable URL: http://www.jstor.org/stable/2713291 Accessed: 02-02-2017 20:55 UT

White, A. A., III. (2011). *Seeing patients: Unconscious bias in health care.* Harvard University Press.

# About the Author

Dr. McAdams-Jones has been a practicing registered nurse since 1973, served as a Major United States Army Nurse Corps in the European Theater and Dwight David Eisenhower Army Medical Center, Fort Gordon Georgia, and is a graduate of Tuskegee University. She is the founder of Justussocializing.net a nonprofit from which she continues to educate on matters of equality. After leaving the United States Armed Forces, she continued to practice while joining higher education. She is a Certified Simulation Health Care Educator (CHSE), a Fellow in the Academy of Nurse Educators (ANEF), a graduate of AACN Access Connection and Engagement, and a Senior Fellow Advance Higher Education. Her areas of interest are social justice and integrating social determinants of health into nursing curriculum along with mowing lawns and fly-fishing curiosity.

www.ingramcontent.com/pod-product-compliance
Lightning Source LLC
LaVergne TN
LVHW060452061126
851857LV00016B/1808